CARDIOVASCULAR DISEASE:
ASSESSMENT AND INTERVENTION

Fourth Edition

By
Mary Stein & Kathy Templin, RN, MS, CCRN

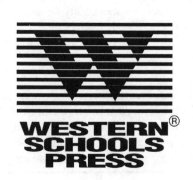

**WESTERN®
SCHOOLS
PRESS**

21 Bristol Drive
South Easton, MA 02375
1-800-618-1670

ABOUT THE AUTHORS

Mary Stein has many years of experience writing for the medical field. She has served on the editorial staffs of *Diagnosis* and *Advances in Reproductive Medicine*, and has contributed to *Perspectives in Cardiology, Modern Medicine*, and *Patient Care*, among others.

Kathy Templin, RN, MS, CCRN, has 22 years' experience working in a clinical setting. She is currently working as clinical nurse specialist, MICU/CCU, at the Veterans Medical Center in La Jolla, California. She is certified as an instructor for the basic cardiac life support and advanced cardiac life support courses. She wrote chapters 6 and 7 of this course.

ABOUT THE SUBJECT MATTER EXPERT

Jean Holliday, RN, MSN, CCRN, is the executive director of Holliday Educational Lectures and Programs. She lectures throughout Southern California, Nevada, and Arizona, providing leadership and critical care information to nurses. Jean received her MSN from Cal-State Domingues Hills in 1988.

ABOUT THE REVIEWERS

Della Burns, RN, MN, CFNP, has been a critical care clinical nurse specialist for 10 years. She has taught critical care to undergraduate and graduate nursing students at San Diego State University and is currently working as an independent consultant.

David Burns, RN, MN, CCRN, is a clinical specialist at Palomar Medical Center, Escondido, California, and has extensive experience caring for cardiac patients.

Copy Editor: Barbara Halliburton, PhD

Indexer: Sylvia Coates

Graphic Artist: Kathy Johnson

Typesetter: Kathy Johnson

Western Schools courses are designed to provide Nursing professionals with the Educational information they need to enhance their career development. The information provided within these course materials is the result of research and consultation with prominent Nursing and Medical authorities and is, to the best of our knowledge, current and accurate. However, the courses and course materials are provided with the understanding that Western Schools is not engaged in offering legal, nursing, medical, or other professional advice.

Western Schools courses and course materials are not meant to act as a substitute for seeking out professional advice or conducting individual research. When applying the information provided in the courses and course materials to individual circumstances, all recommendations must be considered in light of the uniqueness pertaining to each situation.

Western Schools course materials are intended solely for *your* use, and *not* for the benefit of providing advice or recommendations to third parties. Western Schools devoids itself of any responsibility for adverse consequences resulting from the failure to seek nursing, medical or other professional advice. Western Schools further devoids itself of any responsibility for updating or revising any programs or publications presented, published, distributed or sponsored by Western Schools unless otherwise agreed to as part of an individual purchase contract.

ISBN: 1-878025-93-7

IMPORTANT: Read these instructions *BEFORE* proceeding!

Enclosed with your course book you will find the FasTrax® answer sheet. Use this form to answer all the final exam questions that appear in this course book. If you are completing more than one course, be sure to write your answers on the appropriate answer sheet. Full instructions and complete grading details are printed on the FasTrax instruction sheet, also enclosed with your order. Please review them before starting. *If you are mailing your answer sheet(s) to Western Schools, we recommend you make a copy as a backup.*

ABOUT THIS COURSE

A "Pretest" is provided with each course to test your current knowledge base regarding the subject matter contained within this course. Your "Final Exam" is a multiple choice examination. **You will find the exam questions at the end of each chapter.** Some smaller hour courses include the exam at the end of the book.

In the event the course has less than 100 questions, mark your answers to the questions in the course book and leave the remaining answer boxes on the FasTrax answer sheet blank. **Use a <u>black pen</u> to fill in your answer sheet.**

A PASSING SCORE

You must score 70% or better in order to pass this course and receive your Certificate of Completion. Should you fail to achieve the required score, we will send you an additional FasTrax answer sheet so that you may make a second attempt to pass the course. Western Schools will allow you three chances to pass the same course…*at no extra charge!* After three failed attempts to pass the same course, your file will be closed.

RECORDING YOUR HOURS

Please monitor the time it takes to complete this course using the handy log sheet on the other side of this page. See below for transferring study hours to the course evaluation.

COURSE EVALUATIONS

In this course book you will find a short evaluation about the course you are soon to complete. This information is vital to providing the school with feedback on this course. The course evaluation answer section is in the lower right hand corner of the FasTrax answer sheet marked "Evaluation" with answers marked 1–25. Your answers are important to us, please take five minutes to complete the evaluation.

On the back of the FasTrax instruction sheet there is additional space to make any comments about the course, the school, and suggested new curriculum. Please mail the FasTrax instruction sheet, with your comments, back to Western Schools in the envelope provided with your course order.

TRANSFERRING STUDY TIME

Upon completion of the course, transfer the total study time from your log sheet to question #25 in the Course Evaluation. The answers will be in ranges, please choose the proper hour range that best represents your study time. You MUST log your study time under question #25 on the course evaluation.

EXTENSIONS

You have 2 years from the date of enrollment to complete this course. A six (6) month extension may be purchased. If after 30 months from the original enrollment date you do not complete the course, *your file will be closed and no certificate can be issued.*

CHANGE OF ADDRESS?

In the event you have moved during the completion of this course please call our student services department at 1-800-618-1670 and we will update your file.

A GUARANTEE YOU'LL GIVE HIGH HONORS TO

If any continuing education course fails to meet your expectations or if you are not satisfied in any manner, for any reason, you may return it for an exchange or a refund (less shipping and handling) within 30 days. Software, video and audio courses must be returned unopened.

Thank you for enrolling at Western Schools!

WESTERN SCHOOLS
P.O. Box 1930
Brockton, MA 02303
(800) 618-1670

CARDIOVASCULAR DISEASE:
ASSESSMENT & INTERVENTION

WESTERN®
SCHOOLS
PRESS

21 Bristol Drive
South Easton, MA 02375

Please use this log to total the number of hours you spend reading the text and taking the final examination (use 50-min hours).

Date	Hours Spent
_____	_____
_____	_____
_____	_____
_____	_____
_____	_____
_____	_____
_____	_____
_____	_____
_____	_____
_____	_____
_____	_____
_____	_____
_____	_____

TOTAL [   ]

Please log your study hours with submission of your final exam. To log your study time, fill in the appropriate circle under question 25 of the FasTrax® answer sheet under the "Evaluation" section.

Please choose the answer that represents the total study hours it took you to complete this 30 hour course.

A. less than 25 hours

B. 25–28 hours

C. 29–32 hours

D. greater than 32 hours

CARDIOVASCULAR DISEASE:
ASSESSMENT AND INTERVENTION

WESTERN SCHOOLS' NURSING
CONTINUING EDUCATION EVALUATION

Instructions: Mark your answers to the following questions with a black pen on the "Evaluation" section of your FasTrax® answer sheet provided with this course. You should not return this sheet. Please use the scale below to rate the following statements:

A Agree Strongly   **C Disagree Somewhat**
B Agree Somewhat   **D Disagree Strongly**

The course content met the following education objectives:

1. Specified the major and minor risk factors for CHD and discussed the general progression of the disease atherosclerosis.
2. Defined the Health Belief Model and discussed some of the barriers that prevent patients from making necessary lifestyle changes.
3. Described how a healthy profile is developed for patients on the basis of the family history, medical history and current health data.
4. Recognized some of the basic principles of physical examination, using inspection, palpatation, percussion, and auscultation to detect signs of heart disease.
5. Discussed the information derived from the chest radiographs, ECG, stress tests, echocardiogram, coronary angiogram, and electrophysiologic studies.
6. Recognized common psychological responses to acute cardiac illness and those that occur in recovery phases.
7. Discussed treatment approaches for obese patients, smokers, patients with high plasma cholesterol levels, patients with elevated plasma glucose levels, inactive patients and patients with high levels of stress.
8. Recognized the challenges of educating adults about changing behaviors that place them at high risk for heart disease.
9. Described methods for helping patients permanently change behaviors that place them at high risk for CHD.
10. The content of this course was relevant to the objectives.
11. This offering met my professional education needs.
12. The information in this offering is relevant to my professional work setting.
13. The course was generally well written and the subject matter explained thoroughly? (If no please explain on the back of the FasTrax instruction sheet.)
14. The content of this course was appropriate for home study.
15. The final examination was well written and at an appropriate level for the content of the course.

Please complete the following research questions in order to help us better meet your educational needs. Pick the ONE answer which is most appropriate.

16. Are you reimbursed for your Continuing Education hours, and if so, by what dollar percentage?

    A. All

    B. Half to more than half

    C. Less than half

    D. None

17. What is your work status?

    A. Full-time employment

    B. Part-time employment

    C. Per diem/Temporary employment

    D. Inactive/Retired

18. For your LAST renewal did you take more Continuing Education contact hours than required by your state, if so, how many?

    A. 1–15 hours

    B. 16–30 hours

    C. 31 or more hours

    D. No, I only take the state required minimum

19. Do you usually exceed the contact hours required for your state license renewal, if so, why?

    A. Yes, I have more than one state license

    B. Yes, to meet additional special association Continuing Education requirements

    C. Yes, for professional self-interest/cross-training

    D. No, I only take the state required minimum

20. What nursing shift do you most commonly work?

    A. Morning Shift (Any shift starting after 3:00am or before 11:00am)

    B. Day/Afternoon Shift (Any shift starting after 11:00am or before 7:00pm)

    C. Night Shift (Any shift starting after 7:00pm or before 3:00am)

    D. I work rotating shifts

21. What was the SINGLE most important reason you chose this course?

    A. Low Price

    B. New or Newly revised course

    C. High interest/Required course topic

    D. Number of Contact Hours Needed

22. Where do you work? (If your place of employment is not listed below, please leave this question blank.)

    A. Hospital

    B. Medical Clinic/Group Practice/ HMO/Office setting

    C. Long Term Care/Rehabilitation Facility/Nursing Home

    D. Home Health Care Agency

23. Which field do you specialize in?

    A. Medical/Surgical

    B. Geriatrics

    C. Pediatrics/Neonatal

    D. Other

24. For your last renewal, how many months BEFORE your license expiration date did your order your course materials?

    A. 1–3 months

    B. 4–6 months

    C. 7–12 months

    D. Greater than 12 months

25. **PLEASE LOG YOUR STUDY HOURS WITH SUBMISSION OF YOUR FINAL EXAM.** Please choose which best represents the total study hours it took to complete this 30 hour course.

    A. less than 25 hours

    B. 25–28 hours

    C. 29–32 hours

    D. greater than 32 hours

CONTENTS

LIST OF TABLES

LIST OF FIGURES

PRETEST

CARDIOVASCULAR DISEASE: ASSESSMENT AND INTERVENTION

Begin by taking the pretest. Compare your answers on the pretest to the answer key (located in the back of the book). Circle those test items that you missed. The pretest answer key indicates the chapters where the content of that question is discussed.

Next, read each chapter. Focus special attention on the chapters where you made incorrect answer choices. Study questions are provided at the end of each chapter so you can assess your progress and understanding of the material.

1. The prevalence of death and disease from coronary heart disease (CHD) is thought to be largely due to which of the following factors?

   a. Lifestyle

   b. Natural effects of aging

   c. Congenital defects

   d. None of the above

2. True or false: The Framingham Heart Study has collected cardiovascular data on more than 6,000 persons for more than 26 years.

   a. True

   b. False

3. Smoking affects the cardiovascular system by doing which of the following?

   a. Interfering with good nutrition

   b. Increasing heart rate and releasing carbon monoxide into the bloodstream

   c. Increasing the amount of oxygen available to the myocardium

   d. None of the above

4. Exercise is thought to help reduce the risk of heart disease by doing which of the following?

   a. Improving oxygen transport and utilization

   b. Providing a sense of well-being

   c. Stimulating the central nervous system

   d. None of the above

5. Which of the following statements about the Health Hazard Appraisal is correct?

   a It is completed once the results of the physical examination are known.

   b. It can successfully replace laboratory tests.

   c. It uses a questionnaire to develop a computerized profile of patient risk.

   d. It is used for women only.

6. True or false: Anginal pain is often described by patients as "boring" or "pressing" and may be mistaken for heartburn or indigestion.

   a. True

   b. False

7. "High-normal" blood pressure is defined as:

    a. Diastolic pressure 80–85 mm Hg

    b. Diastolic pressure 85–89 mm Hg

    c. Diastolic pressure greater than 90 mm Hg

    d. None of the above

8. True or false: Cyanosis is always a sign of a serious underlying cardiac problem.

    a. True

    b. False

9. What is the best spot to listen for mitral valve murmurs?

    a. Erb's point

    b. Cardiac apex

    c. Tricuspid area

    d. None of the above

10. How does a click differ from a murmur?

    a. Most clicks are sustained sounds.

    b. Clicks are short, high-pitched sounds.

    c. Clicks can be heard only in infants and children.

    d. Clicks occur as paired sounds.

11. One purpose of a treadmill stress test is to:

    a. Diagnose myocardial infarction (MI)

    b. Assess myocardial ischemia with activity

    c. Test physical endurance of patients with severe aortic stenosis

    d. Help obese patients lose weight to decrease risk of coronary disease

12. Dipyridamole thallium stress testing might be more beneficial than regular thallium stress testing for which of the following persons?

    a. Patient who has had an MI

    b. Healthy persons being tested for an insurance physical

    c. Patient in acute congestive heart failure

    d. Patient with an amputation of the right leg

13. After cardiac catheterization, the pulmonary artery catheter may be left in place to measure:

    a. Right ventricular pressure

    b. Arterial blood pressure

    c. Pulmonary capillary wedge pressure

    d. Ejection fraction

14. A type A person has just been told by a physician to reduce work hours to help decrease stress-induced hypertension. How would this person most likely respond?

    a. "I've been noticing a lot of pressure at work, and I planned to cut back."

    b. "I'm busy working on a big project. I need to work more hours, not fewer."

    c. You're probably right. I'll give my biggest account to my partner to finish."

    d. "I'll just take a little nap after lunch and that will help with my stress."

15. Radiographs for complete radiologic study of the heart include which of the following views?

    a. Frontal view

    b. 20° right oblique view

    c. 60° left oblique view

    d. None of the above

16. One way to minimize ICU psychosis is to:

    a. Leave the lights on 24 hr. a day

    b. Move all equipment into the patient's visual field so the patient can see it

    c. Make light of frightening things a patient sees at other bedsides

    d. Warn a patient of painful procedures to prevent feelings of persecution

17. A patient waking up after heart surgery usually is concerned about:

    a. Location of personal belongings

    b. Medication for pain

    c. Incentive spirometer test

    d. Chest tube drainage

18. Why is it important to evaluate all the medications a hypertensive patient is taking?

    a. To save the patient money by uncovering duplicate agents

    b. To identify certain products that may be contributing to hypertension, such as nonsteroidal antiinflammatory agents

    c. To complete the patients records

    d. None of the above

19. Regular vigorous exercise does which of the following?

    a. Helps increase blood oxygen levels

    b. Decreases blood cell mass and blood volume

    c. Increases serum triglyceride levels

    d. None of the above

20. One of the major benefits of exercise for a diabetic patient is:

    a. Promoting a sense of well-being

    b. Reducing the need for insulin

    c. Decreasing glucose uptake during exercise

    d. Rapidly falling glucose levels when exercise ends

21. True or false: Many health care professionals are more effective at presenting health care changes than at motivating patients to make such changes.

    a. True

    b. False

22. True or false: Telephone contacts are often just as effective as face-to-face contacts.

    a. True

    b. False

23. True or false: Research has shown that people tend to overestimate the degree of control they have.

    a. True

    b. False

24. Which of the following strategies will increase the effectiveness of a nurse with little teaching experience?

    a. Reading as many education textbooks as possible

    b. Teaching only one patient at a time

    c. At first, teaching patients who have a common need to learn about a subject the nurse is expert in

    d. None of the above

25. How can keeping a daily log or diary help change behavior?

    a. It keeps a patient's mind off the changes, thus reducing stress.

    b. It gives the nurse a record to check the patient's progress.

    c. The patient cannot share the information with family members and thus does not get immediate reinforcement for the unwanted behavior.

    d. The patient becomes involved in working on the solution to his or her problem(s).

INTRODUCTION

Coronary heart disease (CHD) is America's No. 1 health problem (American Heart Association, [AHA] 1992b). CHD affects more than 6 million Americans, accounting for nearly 1 million deaths annually (AHA, 1992b). In 1990, 3.6 million Americans were hospitalized with a first-listed discharge diagnosis of heart disease and 675,000 with a diagnosis of acute myocardial infarction (MI). Deaths due to coronary disease are approximately 500,000, with the majority of deaths occurring before the patient reaches the hospital (National Heart, Lung & Blood Institute, [NHLBI] 1990). More than 160,000 of these deaths happen before age 65, and half of all deaths due to cardiovascular disease are in women (AHA, 1992b). Heart disease, stroke, and related disorders account for nearly as many deaths as all other causes of death combined (NHLBI, 1990).

It is impossible to calculate the toll that cardiac-related disability takes on the family, on lost hours of work, or the cost to society at large. We do know some of the annual costs of providing medical care to CHD patients in the United States: The estimated cost to the nation is $53 billion. Direct health costs for hospital care, physicians, medication, home care, and nursing account for $21 billion. Approximately $29 billion in future lost earnings results from CHD mortality (National Center for Health Care, 1990).

Despite these grave statistics, there is some good news about cardiovascular disease. If risk factors are recognized early enough, CHD can be prevented in many people. Medical science has made important advances in prevention and treatment of cardiovascular disease. Earlier detection of cardiac disease has resulted in a decrease in the number of deaths. Premature deaths and disability have also been reduced because of improved emergency efforts. In addition, information about the many benefits of better diet and exercise has been getting out to the general public, and there is some evidence that lifestyles are being affected for the good. Physicians and nurses have made a real impact on the number of deaths by encouraging patients to make lifestyle changes to lower blood pressure, to reduce the amount of cholesterol and saturated fats in the diet, and to stop smoking. For example, the estimated number of deaths due to heart attacks in 1981 was 559,000, compared with 540,400 deaths in 1984 (National Center for Health Statistics, 1987). The percentage of deaths from heart attacks fell by about 2% during that 3-year period. Decreases in percentages of deaths related to hypertension and stroke also fell slightly during that period (AHA, 1981, 1987).

The general decline in deaths from CHD has not occured in all advanced countries. Some countries have reported increases in deaths from CHD. For example, Poland recorded a 65% increase in CHD mortality from 1969 to 1977 (Kannel, 1986).

The decrease in the number of deaths due to CHD in the United States has been recorded in all age groups, in men and women, and in non-whites and whites. From 1979 to 1989, deaths from CHD fell 30%, and the death rate from stroke fell 31.5% (AHA, 1992). The decrease has not been equal for all races, and it also has not been equal between men and women

(Sempos et al., 1988). The greatest decline has occurred among white men. This reduction in CHD deaths was about half as steep for white women and for African-Americans of both sexes. This may be due to a number of reasons, including risk factors and socioeconomic influences. The study by Sempos et al. has important implications for health care professionals and underlines the importance of continuing to promote prevention among all groups of patients.

Preventive care and risk factor control appear to reduce cardiac morbidity and mortality. There has been increased awareness of early warning signs, earlier treatment of mild as well as severe hypertension, and better training in cardiopulmonary resuscitation. In addition, emergency medical services have improved. In-hospital care has become vigorous, with better cardiac rehabilitation and follow-up care.

Better medical care after the cardiac incident is only one part of the equation. Another and equally important part has been the effort to educate patients about their risks of CHD. National, statewide, and local efforts to educate people about the benefits of better diet, exercise, weight control, and smoking cessation have played an important role.

Educating patients about their risks of coronary disease is one area in which healthcare professionals can make a real impact on patients' lives and health. Preventing cardiovascular disease in the first place, rather than trying to treat it after it is already under way, is the best strategy. As William Kannel, professor of medicine and head of the Section of Preventive Medicine at Boston University, has noted, the first prolonged attack of chest pain in an asymptomatic person carries a 33% case fatality rate. Dr. Kannel adds, "People who arrive at the hospital or doctor's office after a coronary attack are only survivors of a lethal process that has already taken most of its toll as sudden, unexpected death. Once an infarction has occurred, no treatment can fully restore function to the irreversibly damaged heart or brain. Only a preventive approach in this common lethal disease, which often attacks with little warning, can effect a substantial reduction in cardiovascular mortality" (Kannel, 1986).

In this book, we examine ways in which nursing professionals can intervene to help patients at risk lessen the chances of heart disease. The book examines psychological barriers that may keep patients from heeding dietary and lifestyle changes and methods of evaluating patients, including history and diagnostic tests to uncover early heart disease. Several chapters are devoted to intervening and to educating patients about risk factors that patients can control. Finally, the book discusses methods to prevent CHD in the first place, using as examples several successful community and nationwide programs that are helping people reduce their risk of heart disease.

OVERALL LEARNING OBJECTIVE

Nursing professionals can have a profound impact on patients' lives and health by educating patients about healthier patterns of living, including ways to reduce the risk of cardiac disease. After reading this book, the reader will be able to list methods of intervening and of educating patients about the risks of cardiac disease.

CHAPTER 1

CARDIOVASCULAR DISEASE RISK FACTORS

CHAPTER OBJECTIVE

After studying this chapter, the reader will be able to specify the major and minor risk factors for CHD, and discuss the general progression of the disease atherosclerosis. The reader will also be able to describe how obesity, inactivity, and stress contribute to heart disease and list how exercise and diet can counteract this problem.

LEARNING OBJECTIVES

After studying this chapter, the reader should be able to

1. Specify three major risk factors for coronary disease.

2. Define cardiovascular risk ratio.

3. Name two physiologic cardiovascular changes that can precipitate heart disease.

4. List at least five medical problems obese patients are prone to.

5. Explain two ways in which regular exercise can reduce the risk of cardiovascular disease.

6. Define type A behavior.

7. List three cardiovascular risk factors that can not be altered.

INTRODUCTION

For health care professionals, the starting point in intercepting cardiovascular disease is determining factors that may place some people at greater than normal risk for heart disease. Large-scale epidemiologic studies have detected a number of these risk factors, including hypertension, smoking, hyperlipidemia, and impaired glucose tolerance, as well as lesser risk factors such as obesity and stress. In most cases, patients have a number of interrelated and interacting risk factors. Some are inherited, and some result from lifestyle.

This chapter discusses the natural history of atherosclerosis and the major risk factors: hypertension, smoking, hyperlipidemia, and elevated plasma glucose levels.

CORONARY HEART DISEASE: A TWENTIETH CENTURY PROBLEM

Just looking at Mr. Conrad, you can see he is a walking time bomb. He is 50 lb overweight, a chain smoker, an impatient outpatient who interrupts his physical examination time and again to take yet another phone call from his office. He is typical of many patients you see in everyday practice whose lifestyle places them at greater than normal risk for heart disease. His risk profile is easy to detect. Other patients with more subtle risk factors may also be at risk, such as Mrs. Chaffe, a 47-year-old with hypertension; or 8-year-old Jimmy Taylor, who is vastly overweight for his age; or Mrs. Tedley, a 65-year-old with diabetes who refuses to comply with her diet.

In a perfect world, none of us would eat or drink too much. We would eat nutritionally balanced meals and would exercise enough to keep our bodies finely tuned. We would take time to relax and would avoid stressful situations. In the real world, however, our lifestyles are far more likely to include fast foods, sedentary living, and high levels of stress.

Cardiovascular disease was relatively unknown before the turn of the century. Today, it is our single greatest medical problem, a devastating disease that affects millions of Americans every year. Each year, more than 1 million people have MIs, and about half die as a result, often suddenly. Despite many medical advances, cardiovascular disease, and especially CHD, continues to be the leading cause of death in America. Just like Mr. Conrad, 20% of American men will have coronary heart disease before they reach their 65th birthdays (Keys et al., 1975).

About 65% of deaths occur outside the hospital, usually within 2 hr from the onset of symptoms (AHA, 1992b). Although many deaths occur suddenly, most heart attack victims report having a series of warning signs in the days or weeks before death occurs (Feinlieb et al., 1975).

The prevalence of death and disease from CHD is thought to be due largely to lifestyle, which has changed dramatically since the early 1900s. From an agriculturally based, labor-intensive nation of the early 1900s, we have become a largely sedentary population living in an almost totally automated environment. Although some would argue that cardiovascular disease, which generally appears in middle age, is more prevalent today simply because Americans are living longer, less developed nations do not have the incidence of cardiovascular disease of more developed nations

(Thomas & Kannel, 1986).

ATHEROSCLEROSIS

The heart is a four-chambered pump, a marvel of evolution. It contracts and expands at least 100,000 times a day, sending nearly 2,000 gal of blood coursing through the body. Rain or shine, day and night, this powerful pump, little larger than the human fist, sends out oxygenated blood through the circulatory system, bringing oxygen and nutrients to all organs and tissues of the body. It also picks up waste products and eliminates them by filtering them through the kidneys and lungs.

Cardiovascular disease begins when any one of the following physiologic events happens: (a) something interferes with the flow of blood through the heart and to the rest of the body, (b) the flow of blood to the heart itself is impeded, or (c) the heart's electrical system malfunctions. When coronary artery disease develops, the flow of blood, oxygen, and nutrients is impeded, and the heart, brain, and other organs are all placed at jeopardy.

Atherosclerotic CHD, causing angina or MI, is directly related to thickening and narrowing of the coronary arteries. Atherosclerosis can be a progressive disease that narrows or blocks arteries in the heart, brain, and other parts of the body, resulting in a decreased supply of oxygen and blood to the heart and the brain. Over time, the inner layers of the arteries become lined with deposits of fats, cholesterol, fibrin, cellular waste products, and calcium. Although atherosclerosis is most often associated with disease in middle-aged and elderly people, the process may begin in childhood (Kannel, 1986).

Atherosclerosis was first described in 1915, when a Yugoslavian pathologist, Sergije Saltykow, studied the degenerative changes in the aorta and noted that he had seen fatty streaks in the arteries of children and teenagers. Such fatty changes, especially in the aorta, begin in early childhood and evolve through various stages before becoming clinically apparent in middle age and late adult life (McGill, Greer, & Strong, 1963). The fatty streak is present in the aorta of many children less than 3 years old. (Strong, 1983)

William F. Enos, a physician who performed autopsies on young American casualties, first in the Korean War and later during the Vietnam War, reported finding **advanced** atherosclerosis in 77% of the young Korean War casualties, most of whom were 22 years or younger. The average amount of closure of the coronary arteries was 20%. However, in at least 10% of the young soldiers, the arteries were 90–100% narrowed (Enos, Holmes, & Beyer, 1953). His findings supported the belief that atherosclerosis starts early in life and is not just a disease of middle or later life.

Atherosclerotic plaque, or atheroma, represents the end point of a process that begins when lipids are deposited in the smooth muscle cells of the intima and media of blood vessels. It is also the result of a complex interaction between the cells of the arterial wall and components of the blood, especially platelets. Platelets are the blood cells that are involved in clotting. Lipoproteins, molecules that contain protein and fats, are the primary vehicles for transport of cholesterol and other lipids throughout the body.

Progression of Atherosclerosis

A host of risk factors. No single factor is responsible for the development of atherosclerosis. Although a genetic predisposition may be involved in some patients, atherosclerosis is also modified by environmental influences (Lorimer & Hillis, 1985). Epidemiologic studies have established an association between certain risk factors and coronary atherosclerosis. The most important of these are elevated serum lipid (cholesterol and triglyc-

eride) levels, hypertension, cigarette smoking, and abnormal glucose tolerance. Obesity, sedentary living, and psychosocial stress and tension may enhance the development of atherosclerosis, but these factors are much harder to define. Although stress is often cited as a risk factor, it is difficult to measure. Each person has a different tolerance for stress and may have many different sources of stress. Some family groups have a greater risk of coronary atherosclerosis developing at a younger than normal age. The roles of genetic and environmental factors in such families are not yet known; however, a number of major risk factors can be eliminated or at least reduced (Crawley, Walter, & Hurst, 1983).

The theory about the development of atherosclerosis that has received the most acceptance is that of intimal injury caused by elevated pressure, deposition of lipid, and infiltration of hypertrophied smooth muscle cells. This leads to obstruction of the coronary artery, fibrosis, lipid deposition, and formation of an atheroma, which may then undergo calcifications, hemorrhage, and thrombosis (Ross, 1986).

The first physical signs of atherosclerosis are fatty streaks in the arteries, which are very common. Such fatty streaks appear in children and in both high- and low-risk populations. It has not yet been shown that the streaks then develop into layers of plaque. However, they probably do progress to fibrous plaques.

Fibrous plaques first appear during adolescence but do not increase significantly until the fourth decade of life, when plaque is found in 36–80% of people (Strong, 1983). This second stage of atherosclerosis, development of fibrous plaques, is influenced by cardiovascular risk factors, specifically smoking, hypertension, continued exposure to high levels of cholesterol and fats, and possibly stress. Researchers postulate that injury to the wall of the vessel exposes subendothelial components, resulting in deposits of platelets at the injury site.

The platelets not only plug and seal the damaged site in the blood vessel, preventing bleeding, but also secrete a hormone, platelet-derived growth factor, which stimulates proliferation of smoothmuscle cells. The smoothmuscle cells are normally found in the vessel wall, but overproduction of these cells forms the basis of atherosclerotic plaque.

Smoothmuscle cells also synthesize collagen, a major component of the scar tissue so often detected in atheromatous plaques. Collagen causes fibrous tissue to accumulate, which then becomes laden with lipids and cellular debris. The dead cells coalesce, creating masses of debris. Cholesterol and calcium in the bloodstream precipitate and crystallize, forming an atheromatous plaque. Hard plaques then prevent the muscle layer of the artery from dilating or constricting, and the vessel becomes rigid. As the buildup of plaque continues, severe atherosclerosis within the coronary arteries, or stenosis, may occur. Most people who die suddenly have extensive coronary artery stenosis (Kuller, 1986). Even people who died suddenly at a young age, such as at 35–44 years of age, had extensive coronary stenosis (Perper, Kuller, & Cooper, 1975).

Atheromatous plaque also contains lipid materials, including cholesterol. It is now known that lipoproteins, a population of plasma proteins, are important in the transport of cholesterol. Low-density lipoprotein (LDL) is only one of these proteins. Cells from many tissues have receptors for LDL, so the cell can internalize it and degrade it into protein components and a lipid (cholesterol) portion. Abnormalities of the receptors for LDL lead to elevated blood lipid levels and subsequent development of atherosclerosis. In addition, Platelet-derived Growth Factor causes excessive growth and migration of medial smoothmuscle

cells toward the subendothelial areas. The atherosclerotic plaque may then be complicated by ulceration, hemorrhage, and superimposed thrombus formation (Lorimer, & Hillis, 1985).

Because blood coagulates when it is exposed to a foreign surface, it may congeal around the atherosclerotic plaque, forming a thrombus, or clot. As the vessel becomes increasingly narrower, it is finally occluded by the thrombus. When the supply of blood is cut off, an infarct, or area of dead tissue, results. This result is known as an MI, more commonly termed a heart attack.

The weakened arterial wall may also balloon outward, creating an aneurysm that is susceptible to rupture. Sites that are most often affected are near arterial bifurcations, or branches, where high pressure and flow relationships exist. Smaller arteries, arterioles, and veins are usually spared.

As atherosclerosis progresses, an imbalance develops between myocardial oxygen supply and demand. Oxygen supply may decrease, or demand may increase beyond the limits of coronary perfusion reserve, resulting in ischemia, or inadequate myocardial oxygenation (Crawley et al., 1983). This oxygen supply-and-demand problem usually is manifested as chest pain, or angina.

If one or more biochemical, physiologic, and environmental factors are present, the possibility that atherosclerosis and its complications will develop increases. It is important to remember that such risk factors are synergistic; that is, one compounds another. An example of the synergism of risk factors might be the serious jogger who also smokes cigarettes. The benefits of exercise are outweighed by exposure to nicotine and carbon monoxide. Few people have only a single risk factor. Most have several risk factors, such as a high-fat diet, too little exercise, and personal or career stresses.

Cardiovascular risk ratios. The concept of risk ratio is important to consider. Cardiovascular

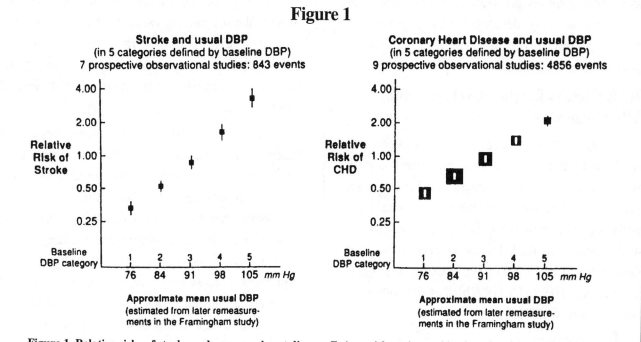

Figure 1. Relative risks of stroke and coronary heart disease. Estimated from the combined results of the prospective observational studies for each of five categories of diastolic blood pressure (DBP). (Estimates of the usual DBP in each baseline DBP category are taken from mean DBP values 4 years after baseline in the Framingham study.) The solid squares represent disease risks in each category relative to risk in the whole study population; the sizes of the squares are proportional to the number of events in each DBP category, and 95% confidence intervals for the estimates of relative risk are denoted by *vertical* lines. (From MacMahon S, Peto R, Cutler J, et al: *Lancet*, 335:765. 1990).

risk ratio is based on the concept that the more severe the risk factor, such as hypercholesterolemia or hypertension, the greater the chances of cardiovascular disease developing. Risk ratios are usually determined from the findings of large epidemiologic studies, such as the Framingham Heart Study or the Multiple Risk Factor Intervention Trial (MRFIT) study described later. The level of severity of a risk factor, say hypertension, is compared with prevalence rates of CHD. The risk ratio decides the prevalence of disease at a given degree of severity by a baseline level of the factor *(Figure 1)*. The ratios developed from epidemiologic studies can be used to estimate a patient's risk. As the AHA has noted, a large body of evidence has accumulated recently that supports the assumption that modifying these risk factors will alter the patient's risk.

Although major studies list "independent" risk factors, these factors also produce a cumulative impact; that is, they work together to increase the risk of atherosclerosis. For example, hypertension may speed up atherosclerosis by forcing more LDLs into the walls of the arteries. Thus, if a person has both hypertension and elevated LDL levels, the two may act synergistically to promote atherosclerosis. Conversely, the incidence of CHD is relatively low in Japan, despite a high prevalence of smoking. The explanation maybe that LDL levels are especially low in that country.

Another point to remember when evaluating a patient's risk of CHD is that the combination of several mild risk factors may produce danger equal to a single major risk factor. For example, marginal elevations of cholesterol and blood pressure combined with relatively low levels of high-density lipoprotein (HDL) cholesterol (a good type of lipoprotein) may be equivalent to the presence of a major risk factor (AHA, 1988). These types of minor risk factors are often found in obese people who otherwise seem healthy.

As described, atherosclerosis begins in childhood. Thus, primary prevention must be directed at people in the early developmental stage, before fibrous plaque develops. Effective prevention should begin in childhood.

Risk Factors for the Development of Atherosclerosis

Study results. Although the exact mechanisms involved in atherosclerosis are undefined, certain risk factors for the development of atherosclerosis have been determined. Epidemiologic studies such as the Framingham Heart Study and the MRFIT study (Multiple Risk Factor Intervention Trial Research Group, 1982) have uncovered several risk factors. The AHA (1992b) lists the following as risk factors for CHD:

- Hypertension
- High serum lipid levels
- Smoking
- Diabetes mellitus
- Family history of atherosclerosis
- Advancing age
- Male sex
- Obesity
- Sedentary lifestyle
- Stress

The Framingham Heart Study. The Framingham Heart Study, begun in 1949 under the sponsorship of the then newly formed National Institutes of Health (NIH), is an ongoing study of 6,000 men and women in Framingham, Massachusetts (Kannel, 1986). These 6,000 people essentially volunteered to be human guinea pigs in a revolutionary study of cardiovascular risks that would follow them throughout their lifetimes. The study looks at the effects of diet, stress, exercise, smoking, and other factors on overall health, particularly cardiovascular health.

Semiannual clinical examinations provide information about the characteristics of the subjects in the study, both before and after the onset of cardiovascular disease. By using the baseline information as well as continuing follow-up, the investigators have sought to pinpoint characteristics that are linked to subsequent development of heart disease.

One of the most important findings of the Framingham study to date is that certain parameters, or risk factors, are powerful predictors of the future likelihood of CHD. The Framingham study has shown that the most important risk factors for heart disease are (a) hypertension, (b) high serum cholesterol levels, (c) cigarette smoking, and (d) high blood glucose levels. Several other factors that were not identified in the Framingham study but were later linked to higher risk of cardiovascular disease were aggressive personality type, sedentary lifestyle and high levels of LDL. All were later indicated as factors that increased the risk of cardiovascular disease (MRFIT Research Group, 1982).

The Multiple Risk Factor Intervention Trial. Another important study, the MRFIT program, was designed to determine whether controlling several risk factors would be effective in reducing cardiovascular disease. Approximately 12,000 men 35–57 years old who did not yet have clinical CHD but who were at high risk because of their cigarette smoking, serum cholesterol levels, or high blood pressure were recruited for the study. These men were divided into two groups, the special intervention (SI) group and the usual care (UC) group. Both groups were followed closely for 6 years (MRFIT Research Group, 1982).

The SI subjects received ongoing interventions aimed at reducing their risk factors. Cigarette smokers were given individual and group counseling. High blood pressure was vigorously treated, with the goal of reaching a 10 mm Hg reduction in pressure or a diastolic pressure of 89 mm Hg, whichever was lower. Participants also received dietary counseling in an attempt to reduce intake of saturated fat and dietary cholesterol and to increase the intake of polyunsaturated fats. SI subjects also had their medical history recorded each year and a physical examination.

Comparatively, UC subjects were referred to their own physicians or usual source of medical care, who were given the results of the screening examination. The health care providers were informed that their patients were participating in the MRFIT study as control subjects. The control group also had annual physical and laboratory examinations through MRFIT, and their physicians were given the results. Control patients received no counseling from MRFIT physicians.

The MRFIT study posed two separate questions. First, can patients' and physicians' behavior be influenced to reduce risk factor levels to a greater degree than would be possible with traditional medical care alone? Second, does eliminating or reducing risk factors affect CHD and, ultimately, mortality?

The results from the MRFIT study were mixed and are still debated. The study successfully eliminated smoking and lowered diastolic blood pressure levels in the SI group. It also showed that moderate reductions in cholesterol levels could be achieved. MRFIT demonstrated that the usual care given by primary care physicians throughout the country can help patients achieve substantial reductions in cigarette smoking and diastolic blood pressure levels and can help them reduce cholesterol levels nearly as successfully as special programs can. The only adverse results came with aggressive treatment of hypertension, which included medication for some patients who might have been treated just as well by diet alone. Individuals in the SI group may have been harmed by such aggressive treatment, particularly those with mild hypertension and baseline electrocardiographic (ECG) abnormalities (Podell, 1983).

Epidemiologic studies such as the Framingham and MRFIT studies helped develop the concept that certain factors could increase the risk of heart disease. Some, such as race, sex, and age, could not be controlled, whereas others, such as diet, stress, and exercise, could be modified.

Major Risk Factors

On the basis of findings in epidemiologic studies such as these, certain risk factors for CHD have been determined. Some can be eliminated or reduced, lessening the probability of cardiovascular disease. These risks can be further divided into two types, independent, or primary, risk factors and secondary risk factors (Foreman, 1986).

Primary risk factors can directly contribute to atherogenesis or precipitate a cardiovascular event, such as MI. Secondary factors do not directly cause atherogenesis or cardiovascular disease but, when added to the primary factors, can increase the patient's risk (AHA, 1987). Hypertension, elevated serum cholesterol levels, and cigarette smoking are primary risk factors for CHD. Diabetes mellitus, obesity, inactivity, and stress have been indicated as secondary risk factors.

Primary Risk Factors

Hypertension

Of all the known risk factors for cardiovascular disease, hypertension has received the most attention during the past 15 years, and with good reason. Hypertension is the leading indication for both office visits to physicians and the use of prescription drugs (National Center for Health Statistics, 1987). Systemic arterial hypertension now affects nearly 58 million persons, or about one-sixth of the adults in the United States and Canada (AHA, 1987). The prevalence is 3–4% higher in women than in men, and the incidence among African-Americans is 12% higher than among whites (Maloney, 1984). The following groups are all at higher risk for high blood pressure: people with a family history of high blood pressure, African-Americans, obese people, alcoholics, and women who use oral contraceptives (Thomas & Kannel, 1986).

Cardiovascular risk increases progressively as systolic and diastolic blood pressure levels rise. Elevated systolic or diastolic blood pressure greatly increases the risk of CHD among all age groups. It has been suggested that each 10 mm Hg rise in systolic blood pressure equates to a 30% increase in mortality and morbidity (Lorimer & Hillis, 1985).

Blood pressure is the relationship between a given amount and flow of fluid, the blood, and the size and tension of its container, the vessel walls. Many variables affect the size and tension of such vessels. The amount of blood flow, or cardiac output, at any given time is determined by ventricular filling, the heart's contractility, the heart rate (largely controlled by the autonomic nervous system), and total peripheral vascular resistance. Peripheral vascular resistance depends on the diameter and tone of the arteries, arterioles, and veins. Unless the vessels are nearly completely blocked from atherosclerosis or another type of blockage, their capacity is regulated by humoral and neural stimulation, also governed by the autonomic nervous system. In addition, humoral agents such as angiotensin, catecholamines, serotonin, histamine, prostaglandins, and aldosterone affect the size of the blood vessels and blood volume (Maloney, 1984). Hypertension can be controlled by manipulating almost any of these factors.

The impact of hypertension does not wane with advancing age and is just as marked in women as in men (Kannel, Sorlie, & Gordon, 1980). Hypertensive women are more prone to cardiovascular complications than normotensive women, although they are less commonly affected than hypertensive men.

The risks of hypertension are also as closely tied to the height of the systolic pressure as to the diastolic level (Kannel et al., 1980). Most studies have concentrated on diastolic pressure as an index of need of treatment and as a way to measure treatment success. A systolic blood pressure of 160 mm Hg or more, or a diastolic blood pressure of 95 mm Hg or more is associated with two to three times the risk of CHD (Castelli, 1986).

When does elevated blood pressure become hypertension? Blood pressure varies widely among people and can vary within each person as well. The Joint National Committee on Detection, Evaluation, and Treatment of High Blood Pressure has recommended that certain ranges of blood pressure be used to categorize arterial pressure in people over 18 years of age *(Table #1)*. Normal blood pressure is defined by that group as diastolic pressure less than 85 mm Hg and systolic pressure less than 130 mm Hg. However, elevated systolic pressure is generally considered to be pressure higher than 140 mm Hg, or diastolic pressure higher than 90 mm Hg.

A diagnosis of hypertension should not be based on a single measurement of blood pressure. Elevated readings should be confirmed by at least two more readings over more than 1 week. The exception would be those patients with systolic pressures higher than 210 mm Hg or diastolic pressure higher than 120 mm Hg or evidence of organ involvement.

The younger the patient is and the longer he or she has high blood pressure, the greater is the possibility of eventual cardiovascular problems (Kaplan & Stamler, 1983). However, problems develop more quickly in older people and at a higher rate *(Figure 2)*. For example, among placebo-treated patients with blood pressures between 90 and 114 mm Hg, in the Veterans Administration (VA) Cooperative Group Study (1972), 15% of those below age 50 and 63% of those older than 60 had a serious cardiovascular problem within 5 years after their elevated blood

Table 1

Classification of Blood Pressure for Adults 18 Years and Older*

Category	Systolic, mm Hg	Diastolic, mm Hg
Normal†	<130	<85
High normal	130-139	85-89
Hypertension‡		
Stage 1 (mild)	140-159	90-99
Stage 2 (moderate)	160-179	100-109
Stage 3 (severe)	180-209	110-119
Stage 4 (very severe)	≥210	≥120

*Not taking antihypertensive drugs and not acutely ill. When systolic and diastolic pressures fall into different categories, the higher category should be selected to classify the individual's blood pressure status. For instance, 160/92 mm Hg should be classified as stage 2, and 180/120 mm Hg should be classified as stage 4. Isolated systolic hypertension is defined as a systolic blood pressure of 140 mm Hg or more and a diastolic blood pressure of less than 90 mm Hg and staged appropriately (eg., 170/85 mm Hg is defined as stage 2 isolated systolic hypertension).

In addition to classifying stages of hypertension on the basis of average blood pressure levels, the clinician should specify presence or absence of target-organ disease and additional risk factors. For example, a patient with diabetes and a blood pressure of 142/94 mm Hg, plus left ventricular hypertrophy should be classified as having "stage 1 hypertension with target-organ disease (left ventricular hypertrophy) and with another major risk factor (diabetes)." This specificity is important for risk classification and management

†Optimal blood pressure with respect to cardiovascular risk is less than 120 mm Hg systolic and less than 80 mm Hg diastolic. However, unusually low readings should be evaluated for clinical significance.

‡Based on the average of two or more readings taken at each of two or more visits after an initial screening.

Reprinted with permission from: the fifth report of the Joint National Committee on Detection, Evaluation & Treatment of High Blood Pressure *Archives of Internal Medicine*; 153, 161.

pressure was detected.

Essential hypertension. More than 90% of hypertensive patients have no specific cause for increased arterial pressure. One theory holds that essential hypertension is caused by increased peripheral vascular resistance, due to degenerative constriction of the arteries. Such resistance produces renal ischemia, which in turn stimulates the renin-angiotensin and aldosterone cycles (Maloney, 1984).

Some people seem to be genetically preordained to have hypertension. Those with hypertensive parents have about twice the for developing hypertension as people with normotensive parents.

Two potential biological markers have been found in children of hypertensive parents. One is urinary excretion of kallikrein, an enzyme that is part of a vasopressor mechanism that keeps blood pressure low (Zinner et al., 1978). Another mechanism is a defect in the transport mechanisms that keep the normal differential between sodium and potassium outside and inside body cells (Edmonson et al., 1975).

Other types of defects in sodium transport across cells have been shown. Some scientists have developed a theory to explain the pathogenesis of primary hypertension. According to such researchers (Haddy, 1980; Poston et al., 1981), primary hypertension begins with a combination of excess sodium intake and an abnormal retention of some of this sodium by the kidney, an increase in natriuretic hormone, and a subsequent defect in transport of sodium across cells. The natriuretic hormone blocks sodium transport, inducing diuresis, but, at the same time, causes less sodium to leave the cells. This increases intracellular calcium levels, which induces constriction of vascular smooth muscle, eventually leading to hypertension.

A high sodium intake has also been shown to play a role in the pathogenesis of hypertension. Although it may be impossible to prove that sodium does contribute to hypertension, in populations with little or no hypertension, sodium intake is low (generally less than 70 mEq each), in contrast with the intake recorded for the average American (150–200 mEq of sodium a day). The average low-sodium diet for hypertensive patients prescribes less than 2g of sodium each day. In laboratory experiments, in animals such as rats that are genetically predisposed to hypertension, sodium intake raises the blood pressure. The earlier or the greater the exposure to sodium, the greater is the degree of hypertension. Two thirds of dietary salt comes from processed food, and the other third is added at the table or during cooking (Kaplan & Stamler, 1983). In addition, Americans now eat more than a third of out-of-home meals in fast-food restaurants, which generally have a large amount of salt in their foods (*See Table 2*).

High sodium intake begins in infancy. American infants consume far more than the 5–10 mEq/day they require. Even though baby food manufacturers removed much of the sodium from their foods, a mother may add salt to suit her own taste, unaware of the hazards of exposing infants to extra sodium and helping them develop a taste for salt that may last throughout their lives (Kerr et, Reisinger, & Planket, 1978).

Another physiologic aspect of essential hypertension is increased total peripheral resistance. Even in persons with borderline hypertension, peripheral resistance is inappropriately high (Lavie & Messerli, 1986). As hypertensive cardiovascular disease progresses, cardiac output begins to fall, and total peripheral resistance increases. As this occurs, intravascular volume becomes progressively constricted. As the degree of hypertension worsens, renal blood flow falls and renal vascular resistance progressively increases.

In contrast, any increase in body mass (muscular or adipose tissue) demands a higher cardiac output and expanded intravascular volume to meet the increased metabolic requirements. Thus, obesity

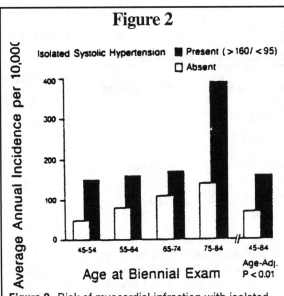

Figure 2

Figure 2. Risk of myocardial infraction with isolated systolic hypertension (>160/<95 mm Hg). Framingham Study, 24-year follow-up. Men 45 to 84 years of age.

Source: Kannel, W.B., Risk factors in hypertension. *Journal of Cardiovascular Pharmacology, 13*(Suppl. 1), S4-S10, 1989.

corresponds to a mild volume overload (Lavie & Messerli, 1986). If the arterial pressure remains the same, elevated cardiac output will result in a fall in total peripheral resistance in obese patients. For any level of arterial pressure, cardiac output is higher and systemic vascular resistance is lower in an obese patient than in a lean patient.

Secondary hypertension. The remaining 10% of hypertensive patients have disease that stems from secondary causes, such as renovascular disease; pheochromocytoma; Cushing syndrome; and dysfunction of the thyroid, pituitary, or parathyroid glands. Other causes include primary aldosteronism, which produces hypervolemia by inducing excess reabsorption of sodium and water.

The heart and hypertension. How does the heart adapt to hypertension? The fundamental adaptation is one of left ventricular hypertrophy, which has been linked to one cause of arrhythmias and sudden death (AHA, 1992; Culpepper et al., 1983; Dunn et al., 1977; Savage, Dragner, & Henry, 1979). This can occur very early in hypertensive disease, and can be seen in about half of juvenile patients whose blood pressure is elevated only to a borderline level (Culpepper et al., 1983).

After age 35, elevation of systolic blood pressure is physiologically associated with increased peripheral resistance, increased pulse pressure, decreased left ventricular ejection rate, and reduced cardiac index. In younger people, the circulation is hyperdynamic, with increased cardiac output and peripheral resistance. Data from the Framingham study have indicated that patients with ECG evidence of left ventricular hypertrophy are at greater risk of sudden death and other types of cardiac morbidity and mortality than people with normal hearts.

Most people have small, variable elevations in pressure. However, the seriousness of the disease can be seen in the following statistic. People with less severe hypertension, or diastolic blood pressures between 90 and 104 mm Hg, account for more than half of the deaths attributed to hypertension (Moser, 1983).

Controlling hypertension will significantly reduce cardiovascular and renal complications. The incidence of stroke, heart failure, and renal disease is markedly reduced by lowering blood pressure. Two studies in particular have shown that treating hypertension reduces cardiovascular complications. The first of these was the VA study in the 1960s (VA, 1967). Veterans with diastolic pressures of 115 mm Hg or higher were randomly assigned to treatment (diuretic and reserpine and, in some cases, hydralazine vs. placebo) or no treatment. The researchers soon noted that complications and mortality were markedly reduced in the treatment group. During the next 3 years, the placebo group experienced 4 cerebrovascular hemorrhages, 11 cases of accelerated hypertension, 3 MIs, and 4 deaths. Among those in the treatment group, there was 1 cerebrovascular accident and no MIs, cases of accelerated hypertension, or deaths. When the differences between the two groups became apparent, the trial

Table 2	
Sodium Content of Some Fast Foods*	
Food	**Sodium (mg)**
Kentucky Fried Chicken: 3 pieces of chicken, mashed potatoes and gravy, coleslaw, and roll	2,285
McDonald's Big Mac	962
Burger King Whopper	909
Dairy Queen Chili Dog	939
Taco Bell Enchirito	1,175
*1,000 mg equals 44 mEq.	

was halted for ethical reasons.

In this same study, patients with diastolic blood pressure readings of 104–114 mm Hg also had dramatic results from treatment, regardless of age. The incidence of cerebrovascular hemorrhage, overall deaths, progression to accelerated hypertension, left ventricular failure, and renal disease was decreased by treatment. About 25% of patients receiving placebo treatment went on to have left ventricular hypertrophy, but this was a rare occurrence in the group who had received treatment (VA, 1970). One area where not much difference was noted between treatment and placebo groups was incidence of acute MIs. Morbidity and mortality were somewhat decreased by therapy but not significantly. The incidence of ischemic heart disease and MI was not affected.

In another study, the impact of intervention was also noted. The Hypertension Detection and Follow-up Program (HDFP) was a large and well-controlled study of about 11,000 people, who were randomly assigned to two groups. The "stepped-care" group was treated aggressively at special high blood pressure treatment centers over a 5-year period. Patients were placed on a strict treatment protocol, with special emphasis on promoting compliance. The other group, called the "routine care" group, were referred for treatment by their own physicians (HDFP Cooperative Group, 1979).

In the stepped-care group, diastolic blood pressure was reduced from a mean of 101 mm Hg to a mean of 84 mm Hg. In those receiving routine care, diastolic blood pressure was also reduced, but not as greatly (101 mm Hg to 89 mm Hg). Compared with the routine care group, stepped-care patients had a 26% lower rate of death from acute MI, a 15% lower rate of death from all types of CHD, and 17% fewer deaths overall. Among people with diastolic pressures of 90–104 mm Hg, the stepped care group had 46% fewer deaths from MI, 20% fewer deaths from CHD, and 20% fewer deaths overall (Moser, 1983).

Thus, the HDFP data indicate that lowering blood pressure over prolonged periods to a diastolic level of 85–90 mm Hg decreases deaths from CHD. The difference of 5 mm Hg made a real difference in morbidity and mortality rates.

Plasma cholesterol levels

High levels of serum cholesterol have been closely connected to increased risk of cardiovascular disease since Virchow's experiments in 1862 (Lorimer & Hillis, 1985). Over the years, many researchers have produced atherosclerosis in many animal species by feeding them diets high in cholesterol and fats (Anitschkow, 1933; Armstrong, 1976; Stamler, 1983).

There is strong evidence that the risk for CHD rises with increasing levels of plasma total cholesterol, as has been shown in worldwide epidemiologic studies (Keys, 1970; Miller et al., 1977; Neaton et al., 1984). All these studies suggest that CHD rates are about equal for people with cholesterol levels up to 200–220 mg/dL. Above this "threshold," increased levels of cholesterol are associated with increased coronary risk.

The MRFIT trial mentioned earlier showed a slightly different relationship between plasma cholesterol levels and coronary disease (Neaton et al., 1984). There was no true threshold level where risk increased.

Instead the relation between elevated plasma cholesterol continued over a broad range of cholesterol levels, although the correlation grew more acute at higher cholesterol concentrations. For example, assuming a risk ratio of 1.0 at 200 mg/dL, people with cholesterol levels of 150 mg/dL had a much lower cardiac risk ratio (0.7), whereas those with concentrations of 250 mg/dL and 300 mg/dL had ratios of 2.0 and 4.0, respectively. Thus, when plasma cholesterol levels rose above 200 mg/dL, coronary risk doubled for every 50 mg/dL increment of plasma cholesterol.

Serum lipids. Of the three atherogenic risk factors, including hypertension, blood lipids, and glucose tolerance, the lipids appear to play an important role (Kannel, 1986). Today, attention is focused on the distribution of cholesterol in the low-density, high-density, and very-low-density fractions. Studies have established a strong dose-related independent relationship between serum total cholesterol and CHD. The impact of total serum cholesterol is greatest in the young. After 55 years of age, little relationship can be shown.

Data from the Framingham study and others have now shown that the relation of serum total cholesterol to CHD incidence in atherosclerosis is associated mainly with the atherogenic LDL component. In affluent countries such as the United States, the protective effect of HDL, is at least as strong as the atherogenic effect of LDL, and this is independent of other lipids and other risk factors (Kannel, Castelli, & Gordon, 1979). Every 10 mg/dL change in HDL cholesterol is associated with a 50% change in risk (Kannel, 1986).

Cholesterol and other plasma lipids do not exist in a free or disassociated form in the bloodstream. Instead, they form complexes with apolipoproteins, or protein substances, and are carried in molecular complexes called plasma lipoproteins. Lipoproteins contain relatively fixed proportions of cholesterol, phospholipids, triglycerides, and specific proteins.

It might be helpful here to briefly review the types of lipoproteins and their activities. Blood lipids (fats) are hydrophobic and circulate as lipid-protein complexes, or lipoproteins. *(See Figure 3).* Different classes of lipoproteins can be segregated on the basis of their density. These are usually separated and classified on the basis of their rates of migration on electrophoresis or their rates of flotation in the ultracentrifuge. Generally, the larger the particle is, the greater its content of lipid, the lower its density, and the faster it floats in the ultracentrifuge (Gotto & Wittels, 1983). There are five main types of lipoproteins:

1. Chylomicrons, the largest lipoprotein particles, primary products of the intestinal absorption of fat in the diet.

2. Very-low-density lipoprotein (VLDL), triglyceride-rich particles produced by the liver.

3. Intermediate-density lipoprotein (IDL) lipoprotein that falls midway between the metabolism of VLDL to LDL.

4. LDL, lipoprotein that makes cholesterol available to cells throughout the body.

5. HDL, lipoprotein that mediates cholesterol transport to the liver.

These lipids also are associated with a number of specific polypeptides, or apolipoproteins, which determine the metabolism of the particles (Lorimer & Hillis, 1985). On an average day, a typical American man ingests about 120 g of fat, containing 0.5–1.0 mg cholesterol.

VLDL particles are much smaller than chylomicrons, about 30–80 nm in diameter. Synthesis of VLDL is stimulated by excessive consumption of calories or alcohol and, in people who are susceptible, by sugar or carbohydrates. Catabolism of VLDL probably occurs in hepatic and nonhepatic phases, just as with the chylomicrons, in which formation of a remnant particle occurs after an attack by lipoprotein lipase. Interaction with lipoprotein lipase then converts VLDL particles into smaller IDL particles. IDL particles, which can be viewed as "remnants" of the original particles, are then broken down even further to LDL.

LDL particles carry about one half to two thirds of the cholesterol in the blood. LDL supplies cholesterol not only for the physiologic needs of the cells but also for any developing atherosclerotic lesion.

LDL is then catabolized in at least two ways (Lorimer & Hillis, 1985). First, a cell-surface receptor recognizes apolipoprotein B and binds it. Next, the LDL-receptor complex is taken into the cell and transferred into the lysosomal apparatus, where LDL is degraded and its cholesterol stored or transferred within the cell for use. The receptor can then be recycled to the cell surface. LDL can also be catabolized by a scavenger mechanism in which the reticuloendothelial system and associated phagocytes are involved. There is no feedback control to the scavenger pathway.

The smallest of the lipoproteins is HDL. These molecules range from 5.5 to 12 nm in diameter and are made up of about one-half lipid and one-half protein. The predominant lipid is phospholipid, next, in order, are cholesterol ester and lecithin. The HDL group has at least two divisions: a lighter subfraction called HDL2, and a heavier fraction termed HDL3. The ratio of HDL2 to HDL3 is higher in women than in men, and it is increased by estrogen and physical exercise (Gotto & Wittels, 1983).

The serum concentrations of HDL have a strong inverse correlation with CHD (Miller & Miller, 1975; Working Group on Arteriosclerosis of the NHLIB, 1981). This relationship is independent of LDL and may represent the strongest correlation between a lipid or lipoprotein fraction and CHD. HDL concentrations are raised by exercise, moderate weight loss in obese people, and moderate consumption of alcohol.

Accelerated atherogenesis and hypercholesterolemia. The development of premature CHD in humans is definitely tied to elevated plasma choles-

Figure 3

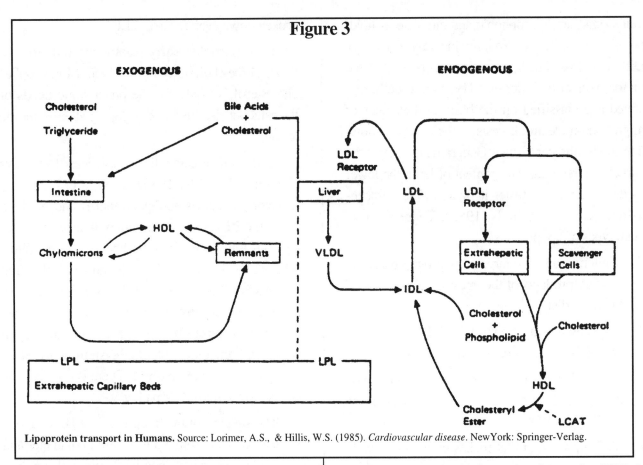

Lipoprotein transport in Humans. Source: Lorimer, A.S., & Hillis, W.S. (1985). *Cardiovascular disease.* New York: Springer-Verlag.

terol levels. As mentioned before, the fraction of cholesterol carried in LDL appears to be particularly prone to cause atherosclerosis (Gotto & Wittels, 1983). For example, in people with familial hypercholesterolemia, an inherited genetic disorder, the average age at first MI is 40 years. In a homozygote who has received the gene from both parents and who has a cholesterol level of 600 mg/dL, a particularly lethal form of atherosclerosis occurs. Most of these patients die before reaching adulthood.

The body rids itself of substantial amounts of cholesterol only through the liver, where cholesterol can be excreted in the bile and feces. The mechanism by which cholesterol is transported from tissues, including the arterial wall, to the liver for removal is not yet known. It may be that HDL acts as a scavenger to remove cholesterol from the tissues, promoting reverse cholesterol transport to the liver (Gotto & Wittels, 1983). VLDL remnants and LDL may also be involved. In this pathway,

cholesterol removed from the tissues by HDL is esterified. This reaction is catalyzed by an enzyme, lecithin cholesterol acyltransferase. The enzyme is secreted by the liver and is responsible for formation of virtually all cholesterol ester in the plasma.

Serum triglyceride levels and heart disease. How do serum triglyceride levels tie in with CHD? Evidence from the Framingham study has shown that serum triglycerides are positively associated with the risk of CHD, especially in women (Castelli, 1986). In addition, two studies from Sweden and Finland have found such a relationship (Hulley et al., 1980; Working Group on Arteriosclerosis, 1981). Others have found that patients with documented coronary artery disease have higher levels of triglyceride than those without disease, or those with normal findings on coronary arteriograms (Hazzard et al., 1973). Triglycerides are adversely affected by weight gain and uncontrolled diabetes, and triglyceride concentrations are inversely related to those of HDL and HDL2 and to levels of adipose tissue lipoprotein lipase. Most cases of hypertriglyceridemia can be well controlled with diet. For example, diets high in simple sugars and alcohol will elevate triglycerides.

Diet and cholesterol. Dietary saturated fat has a strong impact on raising serum cholesterol levels. The major sources of saturated fatty acids include red meats; dairy products such as whole milk, cream, butter, cheese, and ice cream; commercially baked goods; and visible fats used for spreads, salads, and cooking (butter, lard, hard margarines, and shortening). Egg yolk is also a relatively rich source of cholesterol (250 mg per medium-sized egg).

Several studies have examined whether consuming a diet low in dietary cholesterol and saturated fats can protect against CHD. In such studies, it has been suggested that a fat-modified diet can protect against CHD. It is helpful to look at the results of altering levels of saturated fats in four trials, the recent Stanford study, the Los Angeles VA study, the Finnish diet study, and the Oslo study.

In the Stanford study, the influence of diet and exercise on plasma lipid levels and lipoproteins was observed in a group of sedentary overweight men (120–160% of "ideal" body weight) who used either diet or exercise alone to lose weight (Wood et al., 1988). Both groups lost weight, but, more importantly, both also had significant increases in plasma concentrations of HDL cholesterol and significant reductions in triglyceride levels.

A much older study, the Los Angeles VA study, provides some useful data. This was a randomized, controlled study of 846 men living in a Los Angeles VA domicile (Dayton & Pearce, 1969). The men were divided into two groups, both of which used the VA cafeteria. The median age of the men was 65.5 years, and many had atherosclerosis. The experimental group received a diet offering

reduced saturated fat and cholesterol and high amounts of polyunsaturated fats. The other group ate the regular meals at the cafeteria.

The two groups were followed for 8.5 years. The experimental group had a significantly lower rate of fatal atherosclerotic events, including sudden death, other types of CHD, cerebral infarction, rupture of aneurysms, and amputation. In this group, the CHD rate was 31.4% lower than that in the second group, who had eaten regular meals at the VA cafeteria. The overall incidence of nonfatal and fatal atherosclerotic events was also significantly lower, 31.3% in the experimental group.

In the Finnish diet study (Turpeinen et al., 1979), patients in two mental hospitals were divided into two groups and studied with a crossover design. For 6 years approximately 1,000 men and 2,000 women at one hospital and about 900 men and 1,800 women at the second hospital were fed a diet low in saturated fats and cholesterol and high in polyunsaturated fats. At the end of the study, the dietary change produced a sizable fall in serum cholesterol levels, with a net difference in serum cholesterol levels of 15.7% for men and 13.5% for women.

In the second 6-year study period, 1,000 men and 1,800 women were studied in the first hospital and 1,300 men and 1,400 women were followed at the second hospital. Once more, the mortality rates were sizably different between groups who had low-fat diets and those who had regular diets: 53% lower for men and 34% lower for women on low-fat diets.

The Oslo primary prevention trial involved 1,232 normotensive men who were 40–49 years old, who had no signs of coronary disease but who did have risk factors, such as marked hypercholesterolemia and cigarette smoking (Holme et al, 1980). The men were divided into two groups, one of which was counseled to stop smoking cigarettes and to eat a diet low in saturated fat and cholesterol. One fourth of the men did stop smoking, and the net long-term reduction in serum cholesterol was an average of 13% (43 mg/dL). None of the men required antihypertensive medication. The 5-year incidence of CHD (nonfatal MI and fatal CHD) was significantly lower in the special intervention group than in the usual care group. The difference was 45%. The incidence of all types of fatal and nonfatal cardiovascular events and of sudden coronary death was reduced by 42% and 72%, respectively, in the special intervention group.

A more recent study, the MRFIT trial, featured a group of men who were similar to those in the Oslo study. That is, they were frankly hypertensive, hypercholesterolemic, and smoked cigarettes (MRFIT Research Group, 1982). At the end of the study, the mortality from CHD was 49% lower in the group whose high-risk behavior had been altered than in the control group; the mortality rate was 12% lower for all causes of death than in the regular-care group.

All these trials raise the possibility that lifestyle intervention can prospectively prevent CHD in middle-aged men at high risk of heart disease. Medications to reduce cholesterol have recently been found effective when diet and exercise have been unsuccessful.

Cigarette smoking

According to the U.S. Surgeon General, cigarette smoking is at least as serious a risk factor for cardiovascular disease as hypertension and hypercholesterolemia are (Koop 1988). In fact, the AHA (1987) notes that smokers have more than twice the risk of heart attack as nonsmokers. In addition, a smoker who has a heart attack is more likely to die from it and to have sudden cardiac death (death within 1 hr) than a nonsmoker. Smoking is apparently the most common and most powerful risk factor associated with premature CHD (Grundy et al., 1987). Recent information has directly linked "passive" or "second hand smoke" to an increased

risk of heart disease and death (Wells, 1990, Glantz, 1991). Kannel & Parmley, (1986) goes even further, noting that "cigarette smoking is so powerful a contributor to cardiovascular morbidity and mortality, so highly prevalent, so potentially correctable, that it deserves the highest priority among preventive measures to control atherosclerotic cardiovascular diseases." He adds, "It makes little sense to prescribe antihypertensive agents, hypoglycemic agents, or antilipemic drugs to cigarette smokers without making a major effort to motivate such people to quit" Cigarette smoking is directly responsible for at least 325,000 deaths each year in the United States (Luce & Schweitzer, 1978). Inhalation appears to be a requirement for increased risk, because men who smoke pipes or cigars apparently are not at increased risk for CHD (Chung, 1986).

At least 50 million Americans smoke cigarettes on a regular basis. Although the total number of smokers has been declining, because of widespread health information campaigns, and the per capita consumption of cigarettes has declined, the number of teenagers who are beginning to smoke (particularly teenage girls) has continued to increase. Cigarette smoking is a powerful independent risk factor for MI, sudden death, peripheral vascular disease, and stroke (Kannel, 1981a, 1981b). Cigarette smoking is also an underlying cause of pulmonary diseases such as chronic bronchitis, emphysema, and bronchogenic carcinoma.

A 16-year follow-up of American veterans who were smokers also confirmed that about half of deaths due to heart disease could be traced to smoking (Rogot & Murray, 1980). Smoking is particularly dangerous in people who are already at risk for cardiovascular disease and in women who use oral contraceptives. On the other hand, those who quit smoking have only half the risk of those who continue to smoke. In addition, 35% of major CHD events were attributable to smoking, especially among people who smoked a half a pack or more a day. In one 9-year study, death rates from CHD, cardiovascular disease in general, and all causes were 86%, 84%, and 99% higher, respectively, for cigarette smokers than for nonsmokers (Chicago Heart Association Detection Project, 1967-1973).

Millions of men and women have kicked the habit, but given that millions are still smoking cigarettes, the potential benefits from stopping are still great. Some estimate that the death rate from CHD would fall 26% for men aged 35 to 64.

How smoking may contribute to CHD. It is thought that smoking affects the cardiovascular system by overstimulating the heart; constricting peripheral blood vessels; and releasing carbon monoxide, which interferes with myocardial oxygenation. Smoking may also accelerate atherogenesis and arterial occlusion by directly affecting coronary epithelium, depressing HDL cholesterol levels, and enhancing platelet adhesiveness. Smokers also have increased susceptibility to ventricular dysrhythmias (Chung, 1986; Thomas, 1987). Finally, smoking contributes to CHD by decreasing oxygen supply in the face of increased workload, heart rate, and blood pressure (Thomas & Kannel, 1986).

Two main effects of smoking have been incriminated as factors in the development of CHD: the effect of nicotine and the saturation of hemoglobin by carbon monoxide. Smoking high-nicotine cigarettes produces an increase in resting heart rate and resting systolic and diastolic blood pressures, increasing the myocardial oxygen demand. The increase in heart rate does not occur after smoking non-nicotine cigarettes and is greater after smoking high-nicotine cigarettes (Aronow, 1971, 1980).

Nicotine also may produce ventricular arrhythmias. In laboratory studies of dogs, nicotine caused simultaneous enhancement of ectopic pacemaker activity and slowed conduction in both Purkinje and ventricular fibers, making the heart more susceptible to ventricular arrhythmias (Aronow & Kaplan, 1983). In addition to these effects, cigarettes may also contribute to coronary atherosclerosis and thrombosis by causing a rise in free fatty acids and an increase in platelet adhesiveness and aggregation.

Carbon monoxide may be the main factor in causing CHD among smokers. In several studies, smokers were found to have much higher levels of carboxyhemoglobin than nonsmokers (Wald et al., 1973). Carbon monoxide is produced by incomplete combustion of organic materials in the cigarette. It is inhaled along with other components of smoke, which then exposes the pulmonary capillary blood to at least 400 parts per million (ppm) of carbon monoxide. Hemoglobin has a much greater affinity for carbon monoxide than for oxygen (245 times greater), and carbon monoxide displaces oxygen from hemoglobin, decreasing the amount of oxygen available to the myocardium. Carbon monoxide also combines with myoglobin and can impair the diffusion of oxygen to the mitochondria in heart muscle.

Exposure to carbon monoxide from any source is harmful, and the average heavy smoker subjects himself or herself to about **eight times** the carbon monoxide allowed in most industries (Kannel, 1981a, 1981b). Like nicotine, carbon monoxide may reduce the ventricular fibrillation threshold. Other components of tobacco smoke (more than 4,000 components have been identified) may also contribute to the poorer exercise tolerance found in smokers.

The benefits of stopping smoking. People who quit smoking progressively reduce their risk of cardiovascular disease, especially the risk of sudden death (AHA, 1992b). The benefits of stopping smoking occur quickly. When people stop smoking, regardless of how long or how heavily they have smoked, their risk of heart disease is sharply reduced. Ten years after quitting smoking, for example, the risk of death from CHD for people who have smoked a pack a day or less is almost exactly the same as for those who have never smoked and half that for people who continue to smoke (AHA, 1987; Kannel, 1986). A study of British physicians made a powerful demonstration of the reduced risk in exsmokers (Doll & Peto, 1976). When 6,194 British female physicians were followed for 22 years, those who quit smoking added an average of 5 years to their lives.

Diabetes

Both independently and through its impact on other risk factors, diabetes exerts a major impact on cardiovascular risk. Diabetic patients are more likely than nondiabetics to have CHD, stroke, and, especially, occlusive peripheral vascular disease. Atherosclerosis occurs more and at an earlier age in diabetic patients (Sokolow, McIlroy, & Cheitlin, 1990).

Both insulin-dependent and noninsulin-dependent diabetic patients are at increased risk for CHD. Several factors may contribute to the link between diabetes mellitus and CHD. First, abnormalities in the metabolism of lipoproteins (such as hypertriglyceridemia, hypercholesterolemia, and overproduction of lipoproteins) may speed up atherosclerosis. In addition, diabetic microangiopathy (disease of the small blood vessels) of the vasa vasorum may permit increased infiltration of lipoproteins into the arterial wall or may slow the exit of lipids (Barger et al., 1984; Groszek & Grundy, 1980). Increased platelet aggregation may also play a role (Grundy et al., 1987).

Plasma glucose disorders double the chance of CHD in most men and triple the probability of CHD in women. Diabetic women are also particularly at risk for coronary deaths, cardiac failure, and stroke (Thomas & Kannel, 1986).

How great is the risk of cardiovascular disease in diabetic patients? In the Framingham study, 6% of women and 8% of men were diabetic on the basis of a history of treatment for the disease or an elevated casual blood glucose level or glucose above 150 mg/dL on two successive visits (Kannel & Sorlie, 1979). Among people 45–74 years old who were seen over 20 years, there was an increased incidence of various cardiovascular diseases and deaths; this was relatively greater among diabetic women than among diabetic men.

How does diabetes increase the risk of heart disease? The pathophysiologic effects of diabetes on the cardiovascular system are not completely understood. A number of factors have been implicated in the higher prevalence of large-vessel atherosclerosis, which is manifested mainly as coronary and peripheral vascular disease in people with diabetes (Colwell, Lopes-Virellar, & Halushka, 1981). Diabetes affects the capillary basement membrane of all tissues (microangiopathy). It produces abnormalities in the myocardium, major arteries, and coronary arteries (Sokolow et al., 1990). Some factors seem more obvious than others; for example, serum cholesterol and LDL cholesterol are often higher in diabetic patients, and HDL cholesterol may be lower (Glasgow, August, & Hung, 1981). Hypertension is more prevalent in diabetic patients, and more diabetic patients are obese. Prostaglandins and platelet function are also possibly involved. Increased platelet aggregation caused by decreased prostacylin production within vessel walls may be involved.

Another possibility is that microvascular disease directly resulting from diabetes leads indirectly to large-vessel disease by decreasing the blood supply to the walls of the large vessels (Factor, Okuna, & Minase, 1980). Coagulation factors may also be involved in the cardiovascular complications of diabetes, because diabetic patients have elevated levels of factor VI, factor VIII, and fibrinogen. Other possible factors include hypertension and hyperlipidemia; for example, more than 50% of long-term diabetic patients have high blood pressure (Christlieb, 1973).

Thus, hypertension, high serum lipid levels, cigarette smoking, and high plasma glucose levels are major risk factors for the development of CHD. Less serious factors have also been implicated in CHD, including obesity, inactivity, and stress.

Secondary Risk Factors

Obesity, inactivity, and stress are three risk factors that have roots in our mechanized society and lifestyle. They are no less important than the major risk factors, particularly because they can be altered with effective education.

Other risk factors, such as heredity, cardiac anatomy, and age cannot be altered. These factors and their effects on CHD are briefly later.

Obesity

It has been estimated that 40% of Americans are 20% or more overweight (Kelly, 1979). Thus, at least 60 to 70 million Americans of all ages weigh more than they should. Obesity and being overweight and their relationship to the development of cardiovascular disease continue to be widely studied and debated. A number of medical problems have been traced to obesity and to being overweight. Researchers are still trying to clarify the influence excess weight has on the heart, although recent studies point to obesity as an independent risk factor of CHD (AHA, 1992b).

At this point, it might be helpful to differentiate being between overweight and obesity, two terms that are often used interchangeably. Obesity is body weight that is 30% above normal. Overweight is a general term used to define body weight that is higher than an arbitrary standard. The familiar height-weight charts used to calculate ideal weight are most often used to determine whether a person is indeed overweight. In contrast to overweight, obesity signifies an abnormally higher percentage of total body fat.

Obesity is a contributing factor in adult-onset diabetes mellitus, hypertension, abnormal heart size, abnormal heart function, and hyperuricemia, to name but a few *(Table 3)*. In contrast to its direct effects on these conditions, obesity plays a secondary role in atherosclerotic disease. Although obesity is associated with atherosclerosis, it does not directly cause it. Obesity does promote multiple atherogenic traits, including aberrations in lipid levels, blood pressure elevation, impaired glucose tolerance, and hyperuricemia (Kannel, 1986).

Data from the Framingham study provide some helpful information about excess weight and heart disease. In this long-term study, being overweight (as estimated from the Metropolitan Life Insurance Company's desirable weight tables of 1959) was a strong and independent predictor of all types of degenerative cardiovascular disease (Grundy et al., 1987). Twice as many cases of cardiac failure and brain infarction occurred in obese people as in those of normal weight. In addition, there was a modest increase in CHD in overweight people. The effect of obesity on heart disease was greater for women than for men. It lessened with age and was largely moderated by other risk factors. Women had more cases of cardiac failure and brain infarction than men did. Obesity exerted its greatest effect on patients with angina pectoris and sudden death.

In women studied over the 26-year period, relative weight was found to be positively and independently associated with CHD, stroke, cardiac failure, and coronary and cardiovascular deaths (Hubert et al., 1983). It was also learned that weight gain after age 25 years caused an increased risk of cardiovascular disease in both sexes.

Despite the results of the Framingham study, the risks of cardiovascular disease could not be correlated with weight in other studies, such as the Seven Countries study (Keys, 1980). In Scandinavian studies, obesity was a risk factor for CHD only when the waist-hip circumference ratio

***

Table 3
Medical Risks of Obesity

Health Problem	Risks from Obesity
Hypertension	Those 50% or more above their desirable weight have three to five times the risk of developing hypertension than people of normal weight do.
Adult-onset diabetes mellitus (noninsulin-dependent)	Those 20% or more above desirable weight double their chances of developing diabetes.
Hyperuricemia	Increased risk.
Heart size, function	Size increases as adiposity increases.
Menstrual abnormalities	More common among obese women.
Endometrial carcinoma	More common among obese women.
Degenerative joint disease	Aggravated in some obese people.
Gallbladder disease	More common among the obese.
Atherosclerotic disease	Strongly positive relationship with sudden death; fosters atherogenic traits associated with development of atherosclerosis, such as elevations in total serum levels of lipids, LDL, and VLDL; glucose intolerance; and elevated blood pressure and uric acid levels.

Source: Bray, G. A. (1979). *Obesity in America.* Washington, DC: Department of Health, Education, and Welfare, p. 106.

***

was greater than average (Lapidus et al., 1984; Larsson et al., 1984).

Obesity appears to affect CHD by promoting certain risk factors that predispose a patient to cardiovascular disease. For example, obesity helps promote atherogenic risk factors such as elevated serum lipid, cholesterol, and triglyceride levels; increases in glucose intolerance; and elevated blood pressure and uric acid levels. Thus, an increase in weight leads to an increase in other risk factors, which in turn increase the patient's risk for cardiovascular disease (Dwyer & Mayer, 1983).

The relationship between obesity and the incidence of cardiovascular disease decreases with age, especially for persons over 65 (Dwyer & Mayer, 1983). Severe obesity acquired in adulthood is also more likely to be associated with cardiovascular and metabolic problems than moderate levels of lifelong obesity.

To make matters more complicated, different patterns of adipose tissue may affect cardiovascular disease in different ways. In one study, a team of researchers identified people at greater risk for adult-onset diabetes by the way in which fat accumulated on the subjects' bodies. Those who were heavier above the waist were apparently at greater risk for diabetes than those whose excess weight accumulated below the waist. Some persons have increased deposits of fat in the thighs and in the gluteal region, whereas others have major accumulations of fat within the abdominal area. Generally, excess adipose tissue is deposited in women in the gluteal-femoral regions, whereas men are prone to accumulate fat in the abdominal area (Bjorntorp, 1984). Fat in different body regions may differ functionally, because the risk for cardiovascular disease seems greater for obese people who have excessive visceral or abdominal fat deposits than for those with major deposits in peripheral subcutaneous regions. People with large deposits of visceral fat are at increased risk for diabetes mellitus, hypertension, and hyperlipidemia (Krtokiewski et al., 1983).

In 1973, the original ranges of weight for height offered by the Metropolitan Life Insurance Company were changed by a group of physicians attending the Fogarty Center Conference on Obesity (Bray, 1979). At this conference, the average desirable weight for men and women was redefined as the midpoint of the medium frame. The members also changed acceptable weights from approximately 10 lb below the midpoint to about 20 lb above the mid-

Table 4		
Body Mass Index and Relative Mortality Risk		
Body Mass Index	**Risk Category**	**Mortality Risk Ratio**
20-25	Desirable	1.0
25-30	Mild Risk	1.0-1.25
30-40	Moderate Risk	1.25-2.5
40	High Risk	2.5

Source: American Heart Association, 1987.

point. Accordingly, the mean desirable weight increased somewhat between 1959 and 1983, the year the new life insurance tables were published. Weights increased for nearly all height categories, so that the ideal weight for a woman 5 ft 4 in. tall was 120 lb in 1959 and 130 lb in 1983. The ideal weight for a man 6 ft tall was 162 lb in 1959. By 1983, this had been changed only 1 lb, to 163.

Another method that has been used to measure cardiovascular risk associated with being overweight is the body mass index (BMI). The BMI is determined by calculating the weight (in kilograms) divided by height (in meters squared). The relation between BMI and overall mortality derived from life insurance statistics is shown in Table 4. The desirable range for BMI is 20–25. A person with a BMI above 40 would have a marked increase in risk of death, usually from cardiovascular disease. An index of 25–30, on the other hand, would involve a mildly increased risk of mortality (Florey, 1970). *(A later chapter on patient assessment discusses determining ideal weights in greater detail.)*

Inactivity

In the not-too-distant past, daily life was rigorous, and for nearly everyone, work, transportation, homemaking, and recreation meant vigorous activity. Today, thanks in large part to advanced technology and changing social norms, mechanization has replaced physical labor in most phases of American lives. This is true for most affluent countries. Even

sports have been affected. Instead of vigorous participation, television and spectator sports have made most Americans passive participants who are more likely to get their exercise by walking to the refrigerator or refreshment stand than by running down the playing field. Most North Americans get little regular vigorous exercise. There is evidence that this trend may be slowly changing, thanks in part to the new emphasis on health and physical fitness. Although twice as many people report getting regular exercise as reported in 1960, for example, this compares poorly with most other regions of the world (Leon & Blackburn, 1983).

Lack of activity extends to all age groups, too. Only about one third of children and adolescents 10–17 years old participate in daily school physical education programs (Sports Medicine for Children and Youth, 1979). Elderly people, especially elderly women, are least likely to participate in regular physical activities (National Center for Health Statistics, 1987).

In one study, researchers at Stanford University found that overweight sedentary men divided into two groups, one that ran 11.4 miles each week and a second group who did not increase their exercise but cut their food intake by 20%, had comparable reductions in body fat and improvements in cholesterol levels (Wood et al., 1988). However, the men who exercised had no loss of lean body mass, or muscle, which left them stronger than the dieters. The Stanford study is an important step toward understanding the role of physical activity in reducing CHD. Exercisers were also more successful than the dieters in keeping weight off.

There is limited but compelling evidence that inactivity increases the risk of cardiovascular disease and that vigorous exercise reduces the risk (Grundy et al., 1987). We can turn to the Framingham study once more for proof of this theory. One of the components of the Framingham study was an attempt to determine if the level of physical activity could affect the risk for CHD (Kannel & Sorlie, 1979). When people were divided into low, medium, and high exercise groups (low was 25 kcal/kg of body weight per day, medium was 28 kcal/kg/day, and high was 31 kcal/kg/day), exercise had a directly inverse effect on men, but not women. To expend 2,000 kcal/week, a person would have to walk 4.5 hr/week at about 4.5 miles per hour. That is, those in the high-exercise group had less than half the risk of CHD as those in the low-exercise group. This relationship was independent of age, blood pressure, smoking, and cholesterol level, but less than that established for other major risk factors.

Another study, a unique 10-year follow-up of Harvard graduates, traced the health patterns of 16,936 men from 1962 to 1972 (Paffenbarger et al., 1978). Groups were classified according to the hours per week that they participated in sports activities and in stair climbing or walking. When the results were tallied, it was learned that men who were sedentary, and who expended less than 2,000 kcal in exercise weekly, had a 49% higher risk of CHD than the most active alumni. Sedentary alumni, even those who had been varsity athletes, were at high risk if they stopped being active in later life.

In the Harvard study, death rates declined progressively as energy expended through exercise increased from less than 500 to 3,500 kcal/week. Death rates were at least a **third lower** among alumni who expended 2,000 kcal or more a week

through exercise than among less active men. Overall, life expectancy was markedly prolonged in men who frequently participated in active exercise. In contrast there have been studies that looked at men who engaged in vigorous exercise programs after suffering an MI. There was no reduction after 3–4 years in reinfarctions or mortality in the exercise group compared with the sedentary group (Sokolow et al., 1990).

More activity does not automatically reduce the possibility of CHD. Regular vigorous exercise is no guarantee of lack of cardiovascular problems. We all remember the case of Jim Fixx, the marathon runner and fitness expert, who died suddenly while jogging. He had a family history of sudden cardiac death at a young age.

How does exercise reduce heart disease risk? Regular vigorous exercise seems to help reduce other risk factors, such as obesity, hypertension, and elevated blood lipid levels. Regular exercise and exercise conditioning reduce body weight and adiposity by increasing energy expenditure and adjusting appetite. Hypertension occurs less often and at later ages in the physically active than in sedentary people (Paffenbarger et al., 1978). By itself, exercise does not affect total serum cholesterol levels. However, some data suggest that exercise can alter cholesterol levels in certain lipoprotein fractions that are not reflected in total serum cholesterol levels. In the 1970s, it was shown that physically active people have higher HDL cholesterol levels and HDL/LDL ratios than inactive people (Wood et al., 1977). In the Stanford study mentioned earlier, both exercise-only and diet-only groups had reduced increased levels of HDL cholesterol.

Exercise may improve health by reducing other risk factors, but its main effect seems to be directly related to its influence on the heart and oxygen transport mechanisms (Shephard, 1983). It has been shown in animal studies that regular activity enlarges, or dilates, both the coronary arterial tree and collateral anastomoses between the main vessels. In humans, the balance between myocardial oxygen demand and supply can be increased through exercise (Fox, 1974). This may occur through reduction of the cardiac work rate (heart rate times blood pressure for a given ventricular pressure, or improved oxygen transport per unit of cardiac output).

Regular dynamic exercise such as running, brisk walking, cycling, or swimming improves the maximal oxygen uptake. This is due to improved maximal stroke volume and improved extraction and utilization of oxygen by skeletal muscles. Peripheral changes are reflected by an increase in maximal arteriovenous oxygen difference. In studies of monkeys given a diet specifically designed to promote atherosclerosis, moderate exercise three times a week significantly reduced intramyocardial coronary atherosclerosis and coronary artery obstruction but did not increase coronary collateral vessels (Kramsch et al., 1981).

Athletes have lower heart rates at rest and during exercise than sedentary people of the same age do. After a few weeks of conditioning, reduction of heart rate usually occurs at rest and during moderate exercise (Leon & Blackburn, 1983). It is theorized that the probable mechanisms are decreased sympathetic stimulation of the heart and a shift in the autonomic balance. By reducing the heart rate, parasympathetic dominance decreases the amount of myocardial work and associated requirements for oxygen and coronary blood flow. Cardiac slowing also increases the duration of the diastolic phase and the subendocardial blood supply. A further reduction of cardiac work may follow lowered blood pressure, adaptations of peripheral skeletal muscle, and decreased work of respiration.

Aerobic activities such as walking, running, cycling, and swimming are only beneficial if they are performed regularly. Any beneficial effects dis-

appear fairly rapidly unless the exercise continues. In addition, the activity should require at least 50–75% of maximum capacity, as measured by the heart rate. To be effective, exercise must continue for 20–30 min, at least 3 days a week (Thomas & Kannel, 1986).

In almost all studies of the relationship between physical activity and risk of cardiovascular disease, those whose occupations or leisure activities required strenuous physical activity had lower rates of CHD than sedentary people did. Generally, those who were sedentary were approximately twice as likely to have CHD develop as those who were vigorously active. More exercise is not the entire answer, however. Extremely active men in eastern Finland, who have one of the most active lifestyles in the world, also have one of the world's **highest** rates of CHD (Salonen, Puska & Tuomilehto, 1982). Thus, exercise alone can not protect against CHD when a number of other risk factors are present.

Behavior and stress

The final risk factor, stress, is the most difficult to measure. Some researchers have found a connection between CHD and life stress, type A personality, and socioeconomic status, but the relationships are complex (Eliot et al., 1982). By its very nature, stress means many things to many people. Stress is also an inherent part of everyday life for all species, not just humans.

The type A, or "coronary-prone," personality is characterized by competitiveness, impatience, intense drive and desire to achieve, and a sense of urgency. Early studies found a positive association between type A personalities and CHD. However, recent large-scale studies have not supported this association. Specific types of behavior such as aggressiveness, anger, and chronic mental stress have been postulated as risks for CHD, but they have not been studied enough to claim a direct link. Some studies, though, have shown that stress reduction techniques do lower blood pressure and help control hypertension, which may have an impact on CHD risk (AHA, 1992b).

RISK FACTORS THAT CANNOT BE CHANGED

Some risk factors that have been traced to atherosclerosis include age, sex, and family history of heart disease. These, of course, cannot be changed *(Figure 4)*.

Sex and race. Death from atherosclerotic disease is markedly related to age in both sexes and in all races. For example, although CHD is uncommon in young white women, it is a major cause of death and disability in men 35–44 years old. By the ages of 55 to 64, 40% of all deaths among men are due to CHD. African-Americans have almost a 33% greater chance of having high blood pressure than whites. Therefore, risk of heart disease is greater for African-Americans.

Both white and nonwhite males have a higher incidence of CHD mortality, but this is most striking for white males and is greater at younger, rather than older, ages. The mortality rates for women lag behind those of men by 10 years for whites and 7 years for nonwhites. Between the ages of 45 and 64, men have a 44.5% risk of coronary attack,

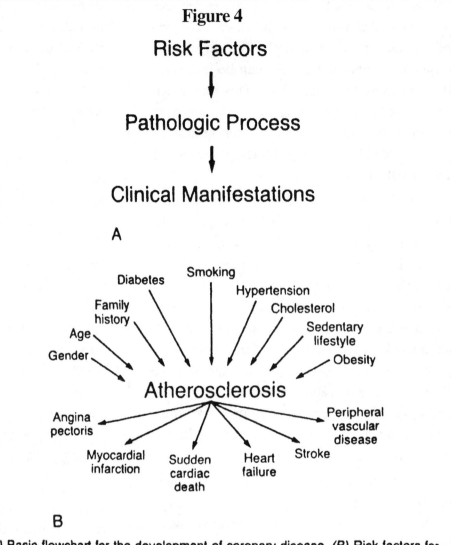

Figure 4

Risk Factors

↓

Pathologic Process

↓

Clinical Manifestations

A

(A) Basic flowchart for the development of coronary disease. *(B)* Risk factors for *(top)* and clinical manifestations of *(bottom)* atherosclerosis.

Source: The Epidemiologic Basis of Coronary Disease Prevention, March 1992, 27:1, *Nursing Clinics of North America,* Susama/Cunningham.

whereas women have a 26.6% risk (Framingham Heart Study). The gap closes after menopause. After menopause, CHD is the leading cause of death among women. After menopause, the severity of CHD escalates dramatically in women. For example, in the Framingham study, women in their 40s and 50s who underwent menopause had more than twice the incidence of CHD as women who remained premenopausal.

Genetic tendencies. Genetics play a role in the development of CHD. Persons who have or in whom CHD develops are concentrated in fewer families than chance allows (Kannel, 1986). Some markers of innate susceptibility to CHD include a family history of premature cardiovascular disease, diabetes, hypertension, hypercholesterolemia, or gout. In the Framingham study, the incidence of MIs in older brothers was significantly related to the MI experience of the younger brothers, even when factors such as a shared tendency to hypertension or hypercholesterolemia and cigarette smoking were eliminated.

A number of risk factors that predispose a person to CHD have been discussed. Once these are recognized and pointed out to a patient, it would seem logical that he or she would make lifestyle changes to eliminate or at least lessen the risk of heart disease. Of course, this does not always happen. More often than not, helping patients lose weight, get more exercise, or stay away from stress is a challenging, time-consuming, sometimes frustrating, and occasionally seemingly futile task.

Chapter 2 describes the behavioral roadblocks that may prevent patients from taking steps to reduce their risk of heart disease.

EXAM QUESTIONS

CHAPTER 1
Questions 1–14

1. The prevalence of death and disease from coronary heart disease (CHD) is thought to be largely due to which of the following factors?

    a. Lifestyle

    b. Natural effects of aging

    c. Congenital defects

    d. Unknown factors

2. The first physical sign or symptom of atherosclerosis is:

    a. Fatigue

    b. Fatty streaks in the arteries

    c. Confusion

    d. Obesity

3. Why is the cardiovascular risk ratio is helpful?

    a. It can be used to estimate life span.

    b. It can be used to detect hidden CHD.

    c. It can be used to estimate a given patient's risk for CHD.

    d. It can be used to predict the need for cardiovascular surgery.

4. Which of the following is a primary risk factor for atherosclerosis?

    a. Hypertension

    b. Advanced age

    c. Low levels of dietary calcium

    d. Type B personality

5. The Framingham Heart Study did which of the following?

    a. Collected data on cardiovascular health on more than 6,000 persons over 26 years

    b. Has resulted in controversial results that are disputed by most medical experts

    c. Involved the investigation of three new major antihypertensive agents

    d. All of the above

6. A secondary risk factor for CHD would be:

    a. Low levels of dietary calcium

    b. Hypertension

    c. Smoking cigarettes

    d. Obesity

7. True or false: Significant degrees of hypertension can significantly shorten life span.

    a. True

    b. False

8. True or false: Cigarette smoking is a less serious risk factor for CHD than hypertension or hypercholesterolemia.

    a. True

    b. False

9. Smoking affects the cardiovascular system by doing which of the following?

    a. Interfering with good nutrition

    b. Increasing heart rate and releasing carbon monoxide into the bloodstream

    c. Increasing the amount of oxygen available to the myocardium

    d. Increasing peripheral circulation

10. True or false: Obesity is defined as body weight 20% above normal and being overweight is body weight 30% above normal.

    a. True

    b. False

11. True or false: The body mass index (BMI) is useful for measuring cardiovascular risk.

    a. True

    b. False

12. In a 10-year follow-up of Harvard alumni (Paffenberger et al., 1978), how did death rates differ between active men and inactive men?

    a. The active group had a death rate half that of the inactive group.

    b. The inactive group had a 90% higher death rate.

    c. The mortality rates were similar.

    d. The active group had death rates at least a third lower than those of the inactive group.

13. Exercise is thought to help reduce the risk of heart disease by doing which of the following?

    a. Improving oxygen transport and utilization

    b. Providing a sense of well-being

    c. Stimulating the central nervous system

    d. Stretching the coronary arteries

14. Which of the following characteristics usually is found in a type A person?

    a. Relaxed and unhurried nature

    b. Absent-minded and distracted behavior

    c. Impatient, competitive nature

    d. Lack of ambition

CHAPTER 2

BARRIERS TO CHANGE

CHAPTER OBJECTIVE

After studying this chapter, the reader will be able to define the Health Belief Model and to discuss some of the barriers that prevent patients from making necessary lifestyle changes.

LEARNING OBJECTIVES

After studying this chapter, the reader should be able to

1. List at least three portions of the Health Belief Model.

2. Name three barriers that may prevent patients from complying with health changes.

3. List at least three factors that interfere with compliance.

INTRODUCTION

Despite all the information about the importance of improving health that we see and hear every day on radio and television and in magazines, newspapers, books, and educational campaigns by healthcare professionals, many patients do not make logical lifestyle changes that could improve their overall health and diminish their risks of CHD developing. They may start a healthy diet and faithfully stay on it for 2 weeks, then return to their old eating habits, or stop smoking for a week or so, then start up again. This chapter presents some of the reasons that patients do not make lifestyle changes that will help reduce their risk of CHD.

HEALTH AND HUMAN BEHAVIOR

It is an all-too-common scene: The nurse has carefully and thoroughly explained the risks of high blood pressure, worked out a diet and exercise plan, and sent Mrs. Malloy on her way, feeling confident that the patient will be able to handle her hypertension very well. The next time Mrs. Malloy comes in, however, she admits that she's stopped taking her medication because she "feels fine." Her enthusiasm for her diet has waned, "because of the holidays," and she has abandoned her pledge to exercise by walking for at least 30 min three times a week. Since she feels fine, she can not understand why it is so important, anyway.

Or, the nurse ponders the dilemma of Mr. Athos, the 45-year-old executive felled by an MI. He has recovered nicely, but 6 months later has picked up his previous lifestyle of working 12-hr days, eating on the run, and smoking two packs of cigarettes a day.

Noncompliance by patients is one of the more difficult aspects of treating and working with patients at risk of cardiovascular disease. It is not unusual for people at higher than normal risk for CHD to ignore or deviate from suggested treatment. One study showed that about 50% of patients under long-term care for prevention of

CHD did not comply with their medications or other prescriptions for exercise and diet (Haynes et al., 1978). The same study found that one third of patients take almost none of their prescribed medications, one third take almost all of their prescribed medications, and the other third comply to various degrees between the two extremes. Even patients who have undergone a serious cardiovascular procedure may not comply with posttreatment advice. Tirrell & Hart (1980) found that more than 66% of patients who had coronary bypass grafts did not comply with the heart-walk aspect of their therapy. *Table 5* lists some of the critical factors that affect patient compliance.

Noncompliance can have a number of serious consequences. For example, a hypertensive patient like Mrs. Malloy who ignores her medication may go on to have a stroke or an MI. Noncompliance may neutralize the benefits of preventive or curative services, and it can also have an adverse effect on the patient-provider relationship. For example, if Mrs. Malloy seeks help and has a number of medications and preventive measures prescribed for her but does not take her medication or watch her diet, her condition will not improve. As a result, she will become increasingly dissatisfied and eventually may refuse to seek further medical care (Woldrum et al., 1985).

In the past decade, there has been a major

Table 5

Factors That Promote Noncompliance

- Unclear or misunderstood communication between patient and physician

- Unrecognized noncompliance by or unrecognized dissatisfaction of the patient

- Physician's ambivalence about the therapeutic goal

- Patient's denial or rationalization of the disease or treatment

- Presence in patient of extreme anxiety, depression, or psychological defenses

- Lack of agreement between patient's health beliefs and the therapeutic goals

- Obstacles to compliance in the medical care system

- Obstacles to compliance in the patient's social and/or psychological support system

Source: Podell, R. N. & Stewart, M. M. (Eds.), *Primary Prevention of Coronary Heart Disease: A Practical Guide for the Clinician.* Menlo Park, CA: Addison-Wesley. (1983).

---

effort to prevent disease rather than merely treat it after the fact. Today, patients are asked to do much more than appear for treatment. They are being urged to take more responsibility for their own health by changing hazardous or unhealthy habits involving eating, exercise, smoking, and stress. Many have made lifestyle changes that are helping them successfully avoid or combat disease and disability.

Under the old system, a nurse or physician intervened after a physical problem became apparent. For example, discovering a patient had an elevated serum cholesterol level would lead to intervention with a diet, and the assumption that the patient would follow the diet. The assumption was that the patient would quickly make the behavioral changes necessary to reduce his risks. Not surprisingly, too few patients changed their behavior, and healthcare professionals were left with the frustration of dealing with "noncompliance." *(Later chapters concentrate on ways nurses can help educate patients about necessary health care changes.)*

Now, emphasis is being placed on patients values, which help shape health-protecting or health-promoting behaviors (Pender, 1987). A value can be defined as a belief that a specific mode of conduct is personally or socially preferable. Values emerge over time as a result of development, personal experiences, interpersonal relationships, and social circumstances. The value that a person places on reducing the threat of illness or on improving his or her health status appears to affect the frequency and intensity with which he or she takes action to protect and promote well-being and health.

MISCONCEPTIONS ABOUT BEHAVIORAL CHANGE

A number of misconceptions about behavioral change exist. For example, one misconception is that knowledge leads to changes in behavior. Another misconception is that having a health motive is enough to stimulate behavioral change. A third misconception might be that attitudes must change before behavior can change (Gutmann & Jackson, 1987). Such attitudes and beliefs may lead to false expectations by the healthcare team and a tendency to view patients who do not change their behavior as ignorant or unmotivated. However, many studies have shown that knowledge and motivation are not enough to guarantee change (Haynes, Taylor & Sackett, 1980). Habit also plays a role.

THE ROLE OF HABIT

Much of American daily life consists of well-learned habits. From the moment a person awakens each day, he or she sets out on a time-worn habitual path, one that starts with the time he or she gets up each day, moves to what is chosen for breakfast, the route taken to work, and even the way colleagues at work are greeted. Some of these habits have short- or long-term effects on health.

A habit is a tendency to act in a specific way in response to certain internal and external cues (Gutmann & Jackson, 1987). An example of an internal cue might be hunger pangs, whereas an external cue could be doughnuts in a bakery window. The behavior that follows such cues may be simple or extremely complex. Cues trigger health-seeking behaviors. Cues about health may come from external information, such as health communication through newspapers, television, radio, verbal cues, or from internal cues, such as symptoms.

Health habits develop in a variety of ways, from innate tendencies, previous conditioning (eating three meals a day, no matter what), and the social and cultural environment around us. For example, a person may have a genetically based reaction to alcohol, but past experiences with alcohol, social demands, and cultural norms also influence drinking behavior.

Habits are also developed from modeling or watching others, experimentation, and direct reinforcement (Gutmann & Jackson, 1987). Thus, most health habits are simply variations on common behaviors that happen frequently. Simple repetition of a behavior increases the likelihood that the behavior will recur. Repetition also leads to overlearning and automatic behavior, so that behavior can occur without conscious awareness.

Habits are often maintained because they have become integrated into self-image and personal identity. A patient may say, "I've tried all sorts of diets and finally realized that I'm just a fat person, and I'm going to be heavy all my life" or "I'm a smoker" or "My family are all heavy drinkers, so what chance do I have?" In such cases the self-label serves as a definition of the person and is extremely difficult to change. Changing behaviors may mean changing the person's view of himself or herself.

Habits also regulate emotions and moods. Routine is comforting. Disrupting routine can be physically and emotionally distressing to many people. A good example is the general physical disruption, or jet lag, that long-distance travelers experience. Eating and smoking serve as easy ways to combat tension, boredom, and depression. Each of these offers powerful short-term mood-elevating effects, despite the more serious long-term consequences. The psychological relaxation gained from smoking a cigarette is reversed within 20 min by the nicotine's stimulation of adrenalin that renews the anxiety. As behavior becomes more potent in regulating and stabilizing mood, it takes on an addictive quality (Gutmann & Jackson, 1987). We all have had friends who started jogging to improve their health and then found that this led to a positive addiction to running. Its addictive quality emerged only when the behavior, running, was blocked, leading to acute distress.

Habits also occur within a social-cultural context. Customs and cultural norms are the source of many behaviors that have health consequences, and patients tend to maintain these behaviors because of the social value. Americans eat not only for nourishment but also for socialization. The Thanksgiving dinner, birthday party, faculty cocktail party, and beer and hotdogs at a baseball game are all integral parts of our culture. Effectively understanding and recognizing the origins and patterns of behavior are the first step to effectively intervening to change such behaviors. To help patients change hazardous habits, nurses need to first determine the cultural and social cues that perpetuate such habits.

WHAT MOTIVATES PATIENTS TO CHANGE?

What factors can help patients change daily health habits? Changes in daily health habits are largely affected by the people and events in the daily world the patient lives in, not by what happens in a physician's office or clinic once a month (Zifferblatt, 1983). Change is a lengthy process that takes years of repeated effort and frustration until the right combination of motivating factors, premeditated or spontaneous,

occurs. Most adults think and talk about making changes in their health habits. Many times they think about doing something to stop smoking or cut down on food, or to start an exercise and fitness program, but usually they do little to change their behavior. Sometimes they make a stab at it and fail.

Any type of successful personal change is difficult because it almost always means changing comfortable old habits, some of which have been ingrained since childhood. Thus, change becomes the exception, not the rule. Changes in harmful habits are likely to occur only when (a) old habits lead to clearly adverse consequences, and (b) the potential benefits of the new health habits markedly outweigh the benefits of keeping the old health habits. For example, a man confronted with an inexplicable spot on a chest film may feel motivated enough to stop smoking after years of feeling comfortable with his habit. Or, a woman visiting a weight control clinic may believe that losing 50 lb will vastly improve her social life.

The Health Belief Model. The Health Belief Model (Rosenstock, 1966) is a concept, based on motivational theory, that a person will engage in health-related behavior because of five reasons: (a) perceived susceptibility, or the patient's perception that he or she is likely to experience a particular illness and/or related complications from it; (b) perceived severity of the illness or related complications and the possible impact upon his or her life; (c) the benefits of action, or the health action's potential for reducing susceptibility and/or severity; (d) the costs of the health behavior, including financial costs, expenditures of time and effort, inconvenience, and possible side effects; and (e) cues to action. The last ingredient appears to make persons consciously aware of their feelings, enabling them to bring the feelings to bear on the specific problem. Later chapters show how nurses can put the principles of the Health Belief Model into practice.

The Health Belief Model was originally designed to be used to predict a person's willingness to become involved in preventive health behaviors, such as participating in regular screening examinations or attending an immunization clinic. Although it was designed to describe health-related behaviors, a number of subsequent studies have shown that it can also be useful for describing compliance behavior during acute illnesses, such as otitis media, rheumatic fever, and strep throat. It has also been extended to help define health beliefs. The following case example shows some of the elements of the Health Belief Model (Woldrum et al., 1985):

> Mr. Jamieson is 40 years old and has been smoking for 17 years. He tells the nurse, "The doctor tells me that I am prone to develop lung cancer because my father died of it. He also said that the statistics show a higher rate of lung cancer in men, and I believe him. I want to quit smoking because I do not want to die of lung cancer, and I think not smoking will help. It won't be easy, but I saw how lung cancer got to my dad. I'll really try to quit this time. Sign me up for the next Stop Smoking Program."

> Mr. Jamieson believed that he was susceptible to lung cancer; that the possibility of lung cancer was serious; and that the prescribed prevention method, stopping smoking, would help. Many other factors also come into play with such a case, such as the patient's socioeconomic status, attitudes about the health-care team, and past experience with the disease or with the prescribed regimen.

Everyone experiences barriers to making behavioral changes. Although some obstacles can not be anticipated, others can be planned for and overcome. Barriers to effective health behavior can arise from a variety of places, including from within the patient, from the patient's family and friends, or from the environment. Some internal barriers to change include lack of motivation, fatigue, boredom, giving up, lack of appropriate skills to make the changes, and a belief that personal behaviors can not be successfully changed.

The effect of family and friends. Social support plays an important part in patients' compliance. The influence of family and friends can be seen as early as the decision to seek medical care, or the decision to work out a healthier way of living. Family and friends can either conflict with or support the patient's efforts to adopt a healthier lifestyle. Family members can also be the source of barriers to changes in health behaviors, particularly if they encourage the patient to continue behavior that is hazardous to his or her health or if they actively discourage the patient from changing behaviors that ultimately will lead to CHD. Family members may be hostile, punitive, or apathetic toward new health behaviors and may provide repeated negative reinforcement for the patient. A husband may resent or be threatened by his wife's dramatic weight loss, or a wife may weary of fixing special foods for her husband.

In contrast, family and friends may be extremely supportive of healthier lifestyles. A study by Aho (1977) of women whose husbands had heart disease showed that wives who believed in the seriousness of the diagnosis, their husbands' susceptibility to heart disease, and the benefits of treatment were far more likely to suggest and encourage health-related changes to their husbands than wives who did not share the same beliefs. Wives who believed in the benefits of treatment were more likely to encourage health-related changes such as regular medical checkups and changes in diet, smoking, and activity levels.

A similar pattern was found in patients attending a hypertension clinic at Johns Hopkins Hospital

(Sackett et al., 1978). When family members and/or friends were also educated about the treatment program, a sizable reduction in blood pressure was seen in a number of patients attending the clinic.

It is easy to see why changing long-term health habits is difficult. As Stephen Zifferblatt, director of the Longevity Center, Santa Monica, California, has noted, "Our everyday health habits are influenced less by health information or by our perception of long-term health results (doing what we should do) than they are by the variables that govern all aspects of our daily lives (social, cultural, historical, economic, and pleasure). In particular they are affected by their immediate and day-to-day effect on our satisfaction and sense of well-being."

SOME PSYCHOLOGICAL BARRIERS

A host of psychological elements can act as barriers to health care changes, including denial, rationalization, depression, and anxiety.

Denial/Rationalization. Some patients have an important need to deny they have a disease or need treatment, or to rationalize its implications (Podell & Stewart, 1983). The disease denial/rationalization syndrome can be an important contributor to lack of compliance. Many patients have some resistance to going to a physician or a dentist, but, unlike those who have the denial/rationalization syndrome, usually their resistance does not pose any huge obstacles. The denial syndrome can be recognized by the vigor of the patient's denial that anything is wrong or by its illogical rationale. An example could be the patient who says, "Yes, I am short of breath and feel faint after climbing stairs, but that's normal for anyone my age." You may be able to recognize the syndrome by three of

its characteristics: (a) fear of disease or disability, (b) fear of loss of a real of fantasized role, or (c) fear of loss of autonomy in the doctor-patient relationship. We are all familiar with the power of denial, as with cancer patients who have been told about the diagnosis yet persist in asking what disease they have, or patients with angina who dismiss it as indigestion.

Depression/anxiety. Other patients may resist treatment because of underlying problems with depression or anxiety. Instead of making lifestyle changes, the patient may be unable to focus on changes because of the overwhelming impact of other problems. As an example, a severely anxious or depressed patient may need all his or her energy just to cope with the ordinary demands of everyday living and may have little energy left to cope with new problems or treatment. Some depressed people may feel that they do not deserve good health. Others may be too rigid to make the changes, even if guidelines are carefully laid out for them to follow. Fear may also interfere with compliance. Some anxiety about changing health may help patients adopt new health programs, but, in direct contrast, too much anxiety may paralyze them (Zifferblatt, 1983).

Other barriers. In addition to the four variables specified by Rosenstock in his original description of the Health Belief Model (susceptibility, seriousness, benefits, and costs), a number of other factors may intervene to block changes in health behavior *(Table 5)*. First, patients' knowledge and understanding of a health-promoting change influences how closely they comply. In one study, patients were interviewed about their medications and asked how they were taking the drugs. This information was then checked against medical records in doctors' offices and pharmacies (Hulka et al., 1976).

The complexity of the regimen is closely related to its chances of success (Neeley & Patrick,

1968). As the number of medications and procedures increases, so do the number of errors.

COMMUNICATION

Failure of communication between the patient and his or her doctor or nurse is another major contributor to lack of compliance (Podell & Stewart, 1983). Clear communication about health risks is extremely important. Many instances of noncompliance can be traced back to the patient's confusion about what the physician or nurse suggested, or to the patient not being able to remember the prescribed behavioral change. There is an old rule of thumb about communicating with patients: In a typical office visit, only 50% of the statements made by the healthcare team will be recalled accurately by the patient 5 min after the interview.

The following are the most common and important obstacles to clear communication:

1. The nurse uses technical terms that the patient misunderstands. Even words that seem relatively common can be misunderstood; for example, to some patients, "hypertension" may seem to indicate a psychological problem such tension or anxiety.

2. A nurse speaks indistinctly, or too quickly, or in a tone that does not carry, or speaks into the chart and not directly to the patient.

3. The patient is given too many instructions without any emphasis on which are the most important to heed, or in what order they should be followed.

4. The patient is embarrassed or too shy to ask for clarification of instructions or terms or information that he or she does not understand.

5. The patient does not think about what he or she has heard until after he or she has left the office.

6. The patient's fears, anxiety, or other emotions get in the way and reduce his or her ability to pay attention to what the nurse is saying.

7. The nurse fails to verify that the patient understands what is expected.

8. The normal process of memory decay occurs.

Why do not patients ask questions when they do not understand? Many patients are embarrassed to admit that they do not know what a medical term means or what a medication does. Others may feel intimidated by a physician or nurse, or even the unfamiliar setting of a physician's office or hospital outpatient clinic.

An important part of the many psychosocial factors that determine whether a patient will comply with medical advice is the relationship with the healthcare provider. Two negative components, which can interfere with compliance, are (a) incongruent expectations and interests and (b) dissatisfaction with the patient-provider encounter or relationship (Woldrum et al., 1985). For example, a patient may think that the medication the nurse gives him or her will bring about immediate relief of cervical pain, while the physician and nurse are devising a program that requires faithful exercise and traction for at least a month. In an extreme case, the patient will become frustrated when his or her expectations are not met and choose not to continue with treatment.

Adherence with any preventive care program is greater when the patient's expectations are fulfilled, when the nurse or physician asks about and respects all the patient's concerns, and when the patient and healthcare professionals agree on specific parts of the preventive regimen. Patients also do better when they think a healthcare professional listens to their concerns, and explains the condition and risks in a way they can understand, and when their feelings about the situation are considered.

The setting in which health care is given can

also influence the success of treatment (Finnerty, 1981). When one physician tried to find out why so many patients withdrew from their hypertensive program, he found that many had complaints about long waiting times and lack of enough time with the physician when they finally got in to see him. The average amount of time a patient spent with the physician was 7.5 min, usually after waiting a long time. In addition, patients rarely were able to see the same physician each time.

Thus, many elements can block or enhance patients' compliance and the nurse's ability to encourage them to alter those parts of their lifestyle that may place them at high risk for CHD. We have touched on just a few of the many and often complex reasons that persons may resist changing their lifestyle, even when it is for their own benefit.

In the next chapter, the focus is on the initial assessment, determining people at risk of CHD.

EXAM QUESTIONS

CHAPTER 2
Questions 15–16

15. According to the Health Belief Model, which of the following people would be most motivated for behavior change?

    a. 50-year-old man who recently had an MI whose prognosis is good and who has lost weight

    b. 60-year-old man who has been obese for 40 years

    c. 40-year-old man who reports that his wife wishes him to lose weight

    d. A depressed patient who needs to stop smoking

16. Which of the following statements about the Health Belief Model is correct?

    a. It is an activity-based health program.

    b. It is a concept that a person will lead a healthier life because of several basic beliefs, including perceived susceptibility.

    c. It was used in early studies of patients at risk of CHD.

    d. It was the foundation for holistic medicine.

CHAPTER 3

ASSESSING PATIENTS FOR THE RISK OF DISEASE: TAKING THE HEALTH HISTORY

CHAPTER OBJECTIVE

After studying this chapter, the reader will be able to describe how a health profile is developed for patients on the basis of the family history, medical history, and current health data.

LEARNING OBJECTIVES

After studying this chapter, the reader should be able to

1. Explain how a family history can be valuable for uncovering risk of cardiovascular disease.

2. Differentiate a preventive assessment from a typical health checkup.

3. Give at least two examples of health questionnaires that can be used to assess psychological well-being.

4. Name at least four symptoms likely to be reported by patients with cardiovascular disease.

INTRODUCTION

Preventing disease and promoting health begin with assessment of individual risks. This includes not only an assessment of the the patient's current health status but also an analysis of problems he or she may be at risk for because of lifestyle, family history, and general beliefs about health.

This chapter reviews some of the methods a nurse can use to develop a risk profile for individual patients. Particular attention is paid to findings in the health histories that are warning signals of greater than normal risk for the development of cardiovascular disease.

SETTING THE STAGE FOR PREVENTIVE ASSESSMENT

Preventing CHD begins with a thorough assessment of the patient, by using questionnaires or direct interviews to gather information about the patient, followed by a thorough physical examination and laboratory tests. The results of the family and general history often enable nurses to develop a profile of the patient's current health status as well as future directions his or her health may take. Some cardiac problems can be diagnosed with a single test, but understanding the patient's full problem usually requires compiling data from the history, physical examination, and appropriate tests. Personal health habits, lifestyle, and the environment Americans live in have a major impact on quality of life, and even the length of life. This is especially true in the case of cardiovascular disease.

A preventive assessment differs from the traditional workup (Sheridan & Winogrond, 1987) in a couple of important ways. In the traditional workup, a patient has signs and symptoms that suggest active disease, and the workup is designed to determine if a particular disease is present. In contrast, the preventive workup measures the patient's current health status and function to determine if his or her current or future health can be improved. In place of signs and symptoms, the age, sex, and race of the patient are the preliminary data that guide the assessment.

A comprehensive assessment provides information that is critical for the following:

• Developing a plan of care that will help the patient enhance his or her personal health status

• Decreasing the probability of chronic disease or the severity of chronic disease

• Helping the patient gain increased control over his or her own health through competent self-care

As other information is added to the health history, such as family history, data about lifestyle, and possibly signs and symptoms, the assessment takes on another dimension. In some cases, findings on the physical examination or results from laboratory tests will lead to a diagnostic work up for early disease. For other patients, known risks for disease will lead to tests in certain areas.

Ideally, the health profile will be developed over a number of visits because of the obvious amount of time it takes to do a comprehensive evaluation and to compile personal data. During the first visit, the nurse can give the client an overview of the areas that will be evaluated during subsequent visits (Pender, 1987). This will give the patient a chance to be better prepared to give the nurse more specific information, for example, about the number and relationship of relatives who have had CHD. Scheduling more than one session also will help the client feel more comfortable with

the nurse and more at ease sharing lifestyle information. Stressing that such information will be confidential and used only for designing a health improvement plan (if needed) will also put the patient at greater ease.

Some have suggested that the preventive assessment be performed in the patient's home (Pender, 1987), because this provides a non-threatening setting. It also allows the nurse to see patients in their own natural home setting and to observe their physical and family environment. All these things may give clues to CHD risks that might not occur to the patient or the nurse in a clinical setting.

During the health assessment, it is important to create a feeling of unconditional, nonjudgmental acceptance. A supportive, empathetic, professional, and nonjudgmental attitude will create a better climate, one that will produce a better health profile. If patients feel they will be censored or judged because of parts of their lifestyle, they most likely will leave out such information. An example is the woman who drinks too much but is too ashamed to mention her increasing problem with alcohol. In the right setting, she may be more likely to share the information about her addiction to alcohol, and thus have a better chance for getting help.

The nurse can also tailor the assessment more closely to the individual by considering three questions:

1. Are the health and history questions appropriate for this patient?

2. What is the quality of the information being gathered?

3. What is the cost of gathering the information?

For example, it is probably not relevant to ask Scandinavians about a family history of sickle cell disease, whereas it is an appropriate and essential question for a young African-American couple considering having a baby (Sheridan & Winogrond, 1987). Ordering laboratory tests is another way of assessing health and may or may not be appropriate, depending on the individual case.

The Canadian Task Force on the Periodic Health Examination has defined the conditions that are appropriate for periodic assessment (1979). The following criteria for tests takes into account the attributes of the condition, the availability of a test for it, and the suitability of testing for it. These are the criteria:

1. The condition generates a significant burden or suffering for the person (consider: years of life lost; the degree of disability, pain, and discomfort; cost of treatment; or effect on the family) or for society (loss of productive years, loss of taxable income, or cost of treatment). In addition, the condition must have an effective treatment that can reduce the risk of the condition or the burden of suffering from that incurred if the disease is diagnosed in a symptomatic stage (attributes of the condition).

2. There is a procedure, such as a history, physical examination, or laboratory test, that is both valid (sensitive and specific) and acceptable (patients comfort, minimal complications, relatively inexpensive) that can be used to determine the risk of the early asymptomatic stage of the condition (attributes of the test).

3. Criteria can be established for applying the test to particular persons for whom the benefits of performing the test outweigh the costs involved. The criteria should indicate to whom the test should be applied and how often it should be done (application of the test).

THE HEALTH HISTORY ASSESSMENT

A complete health history, including a family health history, is the first step in the preventive assessment. Careful history taking is one of the most vital contributions a nurse can make to a patient, particularly a patient who has a cardiovascular problem. The assessment helps to pinpoint the source of the problem and provides a baseline against which to measure effectiveness of treatment. In the rush to determine a patient's problem, the nurse may be tempted to overlook the medical history. However, the information that patients give may be crucial (Breu, 1987).

There are many history forms, and a hospital or office may have a general questionnaire that is filled in by both the nurse and the patient or mailed to the patient to complete before the first office visit. In addition, a number of questions about stress and lifestyle may be asked on separate forms or during subsequent interviews.

The goals of individual and family medical histories are as follows:

1. To establish rapport with the patient.

2. To obtain diagnostic information about the patient; determine the severity of the problem; and find other sources of information, including the names of other physicians who have treated the patient in the past.

3. To assess the patient's personality traits.

4. To assess the patient's level of understanding.

5. To assess the patient's personal goals and requirements concerning suggested lifestyle and health-promoting changes.

Health History

A typical health history, whether obtained by questionnaire or by interview, usually contains the following components:

- Name of patient
- Patient's address
- Patient's telephone number
- Name of patient's private physician
- Patient's place of employment
- Demographic data: age, occupation, marital status, education, religion, and race
- Source of referral (if any)
- Date of history
- Source of history (patient or relative if patient is impaired)
- Chief complaint, if any: a description, in the patient's own words, of the nature and duration of the health problem or problems

Description of Present Illness or Illnesses, If Any

Patients give a chronologic description of their current health problem or problems. They describe the initial onset of the problem, the setting in which it occurred, and if it recurred or was exacerbated by another problem or disease. Each sign and symptom is described by its location, quality, severity, onset, duration, frequency, and the factors that seem to aggravate it or to soothe it. Risk factors or family history should be included.

Previous Medical History

- Childhood illnesses
- Immunizations (tetanus, pertussis, diphtheria, measles, polio, German measles, mumps, influenza, pneumonia)
- Major adult illnesses
- Operations
- Injuries
- Visits to an emergency department
- Hospitalizations, if not already described
- Obstetric history (if applicable)
- All current medications being used, includ-

ing home remedies

- Use of coffee, alcohol, other drugs, and tobacco
- Allergies or sensitivities to drugs

Family History and Genetic Information

- Ages and health or cause of death of immediate family members (spouse, parents, siblings, children, and grandparents), if known.
- Chronic health conditions in members of immediate family, for example, diabetes, **heart disease, hypertension, stroke,** renal disease, cancer, arthritis, anemia, headaches, nervous disorders, mental illness, or any signs and symptoms like those the patient is experiencing

Psychosocial History

- Date of birth and places of residence
- Family structure
- Educational history
- Significant experiences during childhood and adolescence
- Marital history
- Home situation
- Significant others and support systems
- Religious and cultural beliefs that affect perceptions of health, illness, and health care
- Job history
- Travel and military history (if applicable)
- Use of leisure time
- Financial status
- Sources of satisfaction and distress
- Profile of a typical day: activity, diet, sleep, recreation, and social activities
- Lifestyle and health habits (assessed separately)

Review of Body Systems

General information: Usual weight, any recent weight change, weakness, fatigue, fever, chills, dizziness, sweating, anorexia

Skin: Any rashes, lumps, itching, dryness, color changes, changes in pigmented areas, changes in the hair or nails

Neurologic system: Headaches, head injury, syncope, fainting, lack of coordination, seizures, paralysis, local weakness, numbness, tingling, tremors, pain, or unusual reactions to heat or cold

Eyes: Vision corrected by glasses or contact lenses? Date of last eye examination, pain, redness, excessive tearing, double vision, halos around lights, color blindness, night blindness, photophobia

Nose and sinuses: Frequent colds, nasal congestion, chronic discharge, obstruction, hay fever, nosebleeds, sinus pain

Mouth and throat: General condition of teeth and gums, date of last dental examination, sore tongue, frequent sore throat, hoarseness

Neck: Lumps, swollen glands, goiter, restricted motion

Breasts: Self-examination? Lumps, pain, nipple discharge, swelling, asymmetry, dimpling, trauma, date of last mammogram (if applicable)

Respiratory system: Cough, excessive sputum, hemoptysis, wheezing, asthma, bronchitis, emphysema, tuberculosis, tuberculin test, last chest rediograph

Cardiovascular system: Palpitations, chest pain, heart murmurs, dyspnea, orthopnea, paroxysmal dyspnea, peripheral edema, cyanosis, hypertension, varicose veins, intermittent claudication, thrombophlebitis

Gastrointestinal system: Trouble swallowing, heartburn, belching, bloating, food intolerance, nausea, vomiting, hematemesis, indigestion, change in bowel habits, rectal bleeding or black tarry stools, constipation, diarrhea, abdominal pain, hemorrhoids, jaundice, liver or gallbladder trouble, hepatitis

Urinary: Frequency of urination, polyuria, nocturia, dysuria, hematuria, urgency, hesitancy, incontinence, penile discharge, force of stream, passage of stones or "gravel"

Genitourinary-reproductive system:

Males: Hernias, scrotal pain or masses, frequency of intercourse, impotence, premature ejaculation, history of venereal disease

Females: Age at onset of menstruation; regularity, frequency, and length of menstrual periods; amount of bleeding; bleeding between periods or after intercourse; last menstrual period; dysmenorrhea; amenorrhea; age at menopause; postmenopausal difficulties (if any); last Pap smear; frequency of intercourse; birth-control methods (if applicable); any itching or discharge; frigidity or difficulties with orgasm

Musculoskeletal system: Limitation of movement, trauma, pain, heat, redness, tenderness, swelling or crepitus of joints, backache, muscle pains or cramps

Lymph nodes: Enlargement, pain

Endocrine system: Goiter, exophthalmia, excessive sweating, excessive thirst, excessive hunger, polyuria, glycosuria, changes in secondary sex characteristics

Psychiatric: Depression, hostility, apathy, phobias, nervousness

ASSESSING A PATIENT'S RISK

Several patient history questionnaires and interview questions have been developed to help health care professionals determine a person's risk for cardiovascular disease. These are then paired with the results of the physical examination and laboratory tests to develop a risk profile.

One of the best-known questionnaires is the Health Hazard Appraisal (HHA), developed in 1970 by Lewis C. Robbins and Jack C. Hall, at Indiana University School of Medicine, Indianapolis. These cardiologists used actuarial data on the natural history of disease to develop a computerized questionnaire that could be individualized to each patient, for age, sex, and race. This questionnaire was developed to determine the patient's total risk of disease and death, to search out new risks, and to intervene with changes in lifestyle before disease and injury occurred (Hall, 1980).

The HHA uses a 48-question history form and measurements of blood pressure and cholesterol as a basis for estimating the patient's chances for the development of diseases that are most likely to strike people in the same age-sex-race group. Typical questions might include the following: "Is your natural mother alive?" or "If she is dead, did she die of heart disease?" or "Have you ever been told that you have diabetes (too much sugar in the blood)?"

Figure 5

Health Hazard Appraisal Form

METHODIST HOSPITAL PROSPECTIVE MEDICINE — PATIENT NO. 297-28-8923
PROCESSED FOR· DEPAUW FAC — INEII 03/08/79

NAME: EDDIE, FAST — WEIGHT: 160 IDEAL: 143
999 S SWIFT — HEIGHT: 68 INCHES
GREENCASTLE IN 46135 — BIRTHDATE: 03/30/30
RACE: WHITE SEX: MALE — AGE: 48 YEARS
BLOOD PRESSURE: 140/100 — CHOLESTEROL: 248

OUR APPRAISAL SHOWS THAT THE AVERAGE RISK FOR INDIVIDUALS OF YOUR SEX, RACE AND AGE GROUP IS 8,298 DEATHS PER 100,000 INDIVIDUALS OVER THE NEXT TEN YEARS. HOWEVER, WE FIND THAT YOUR SPECIFIC RISKS PLACE YOU IN A GROUP WHICH WOULD HAVE 16,770 DEATHS PER 100,000 INDIVIDUALS, GIVING YOU AN APPRAISAL AGE OF 55.6 YEARS.

THERE ARE THESE WAYS, HOWEVER, THAT YOU CAN REDUCE YOUR APPRAISAL AGE.

- IF YOU ADHERE TO AN EXERCISE PROGRAM AS PRESCRIBED BY YOUR DOCTOR YOUR RISK OF DYING FROM HEART DISEASE WILL BE REDUCED . 4.3 YEARS
- IF YOU REDUCE YOUR BLOOD PRESSURE WITH DIET AND/OR DRUGS AT THE RECOMMENDATION OF YOUR DOCTOR, YOUR RISK OF DYING FROM HEART DISEASE AND STROKES WILL BE REDUCED.................. 2.9 YEARS
- IF YOU STOP DRINKING ALCOHOL COMPLETELY OR DO NOT DRIVE AFTER DRINKING OR RIDE WITH SOMEONE WHO HAS BEEN DRINKING YOUR RISK OF DYING FROM MOTOR VEHICLE ACCIDENTS, CIRRHOSIS OF THE LIVER, AND PNEUMONIA WILL BE REDUCED........................ 1.4 YEARS
- IF YOU REDUCE YOUR BLOOD FATS (CHOLESTEROL) WITH DIET AND/OR DRUGS AT THE RECOMMENDATION OF YOUR DOCTOR, YOUR RISK OF DYING FROM HEART DISEASE AND STROKES WILL BE REDUCED......... 0.6 YEARS
- IF YOU DO NOT USE ANY DRUGS OR MEDICATION BEFORE DRIVING UNLESS YOU HAVE CONSULTED YOUR DOCTOR, YOUR RISK OF DYING FROM MOTOR VEHICLE ACCIDENTS WILL BE REDUCED...................... 0.1 YEARS
- IF YOU HAVE A YEARLY PROCTOSIGMOIDOSCOPY(RECTAL EXAMINATION), OF 3 NEGATIVE TESTS FOR COLON BLEEDING, YOUR RISK OF DYING FROM CANCER OF THE RECTUM WILL BE REDUCED.................. 0.1 YEARS
- IF YOU WEAR SEAT BELTS ALL OF THE TIME, YOUR RISK OF DYING FROM MOTOR VEHICLE ACCIDENTS WILL BE REDUCED............... 0.1 YEARS
- IF YOU CONTINUE TO NOT SMOKE, YOUR RISK OF DYING FROM HEART DISEASE AND LUNG CANCER WILL BE REDUCED................ 0.1 YEARS
- IF YOU HAVE NOT ANSWERED ALL QUESTIONS TRUTHFULLY OR HAVE HAD PREVIOUS PROBLEMS WITH HEART ATTACKS, STROKES, ETC., YOUR APPRAISAL WILL NOT ACCURATELY REFLECT YOUR USEFUL LIFE EXPECTANCY THIS APPRAISAL IS BASED ON INFORMATION YOU HAVE SUPPLIED THE FOLLOWING ILLNESS(ES) COULD SERIOUSLY EFFECT YOUR USEFUL LIFE EXPECTANCY. WE RECOMMEND THAT YOU SEE YOUR PHYSICIAN FOR THESE...

MEDICATION USED FOR HIGH BLOOD PRESSURE.

H.H.A. STRESS
HIGH STRESS AND CHANCE OF ILLNESS

SOME RESPECTED MEDICAL SCIENTISTS SUGGEST YOUR AFFIRMATIVE ANSWERS TO CHANGES OR STRESSORS IN YOUR LIFE INDICATE THE CHANGES ARE IN SUFFICIENT AMOUNT THAT YOU STAND A 50-50 CHANCE OF SUSTAINING A SERIOUS ILLNESS, INJURY OR ACCIDENT IN THE NEXT YEAR.

YOU MAY DECREASE YOUR RISK BY FINDING ACCEPTABLE DIVERSIONS FROM WHATEVER IS WORRISOME OR STRESSFUL TO YOU.

SELF-OBSERVABLE SIGNS OR SIGNALS [illegible] IMPENDING ILLNESS, INJURY OR ACCIDENT ARE: INABILITY TO SLEEP, [illegible] EXCESSIVE APPETITE, GENERAL IRRITABI[illegible] FEELING [illegible] URGE TO CRY EASILY,

Source: Hall, J. C. (1980). The case for health hazard appraisals: Which health-screening techniques are cost-effective? *Diagnosis*, 2, 60-82.

The questionnaire also asks a number of questions about lifestyle, including ones about the use of seat belts and life stresses.

After the answers are tallied, the computerized program develops a risk profile tailored to the patient. The HHA also can be used as a tool to help educate patients about their risks. For example, as shown in *Figure 5*, the reduction of risk as a result of positive health actions is shown. Thus, a patient such as the fictitious one portrayed in *Figure 5* would have a reduced risk of death from heart disease if he adhered to an exercise program suggested by his physician.

Many physicians and nurses prefer to mail patients a questionnaire to be completed before the initial session. A completed questionnaire helps determine the patient's concerns and is a time-saving and cost-effective method to help direct the interview. The information is also helpful for targeting the physical examination and tests to specific areas of risk and concern. Patients also have more time to think about answering individual questions and may be able to have the input of family or spouse.

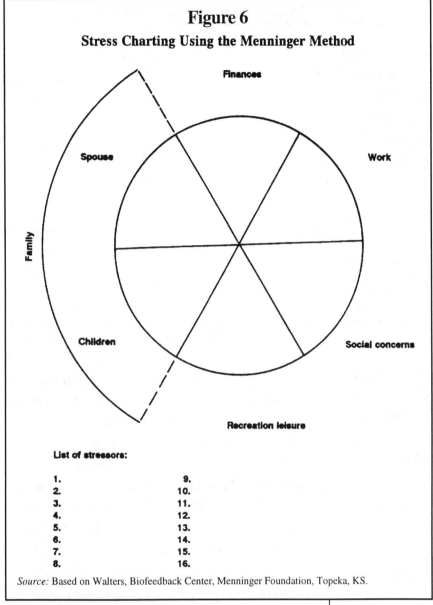

Figure 6

Stress Charting Using the Menninger Method

Finances

Spouse

Work

Family

Children

Social concerns

Recreation leisure

List of stressors:

1.	9.
2.	10.
3.	11.
4.	12.
5.	13.
6.	14.
7.	15.
8.	16.

Source: Based on Walters, Biofeedback Center, Menninger Foundation, Topeka, KS.

Menninger Clinic (Walters, 1980).

These tests help determine how the patient perceives his or her health, especially in relation to other people (Pender, 1987). The answers may give clues about what patients value most about their health and where they would like to improve their health. It is also helpful to try to determine what control patients feel they have over their own health and how motivated they might be to try to improve their health.

Along with the general medical history, it is helpful to develop a history of intake of substances that may affect overall health. The results will be better and more complete results if questions about substance use are phrased so that they do not sound judgmental. For example, the topic of alcohol use or use of other substances can be introduced by including a question in the family history, for example, by asking whether any family member has had a drinking problem or a problem with other types of substances. If the patient does drink, questions about when drinking began, the frequency, and amount, and any adverse consequences of early drinking are usually answered honestly because they are less threatening than questions about "current drinking patterns." By asking, "How much do you drink at one time?" the nurse can often get a more accurate response than by asking, "How much do you drink?" (Pender, 1987).

The CAGE (an acronym for cut, annoyed, guilty, eye) questionnaire, can help determine if drinking behavior is causing problems and can set the stage for talking about the problems with the

Beyond the general health profile, a number of tests and questionnaires, such as the CAGE questions for suspected alcoholism (Ewing, 1984), the Family APGAR (Smilkstein, Ashworth & Montano, 1982), and the Life Satisfaction Index (Wood, 1969), are available for uncovering problems with substance abuse, life stresses, psychological satisfaction, and self-esteem. Instruments for measuring life stresses include: the Life-Change Index (Holmes & Rahe, 1967), the State-Trait Anxiety Inventory (Spielberger, 1970), the Signs of Distress (Everly & Girdano, 1980), and the Stress Charting method *(Figure 6)* developed at the patient. The questionnaire contains the following four questions:

1. Have you every felt the need to Cut down your drinking?

2. Have you ever felt Annoyed by criticism of your drinking?

3. Have you had Guilty feelings about drinking?

4. Do you ever take a morning Eye-opener?

An affirmative or even an evasive answer to these questions then opens the door to further discussion, and to confronting the problem directly.

The Family APGAR (an acronym for adaptation, partnership, growth, affection, and resolve) allows patients to answer five questions about their family and/or friends and provides a nonthreatening way for patients to comment about their satisfaction with persons close to them. The answers are scored from 0 to 2, so that a score higher than 10 signals possible problems.

A typical question with three possible responses is as follows:

1. I find that my family accepts my wishes to take on new activities or make changes in my lifestyle:

   (a) Hardly ever

   (b) Some of the time

   (c) Most of the time

The Life-Change Index is another tool to measure the impact of life changes as a predictor of illness. If enough changes occur within a 2-year period, the chances of an illness developing are often increased. Stressful life events often seem to precede many health problems, such as CHD, accidents, and perhaps even malignant disease. *Table 6* lists several stressful life events and the scale of impact for each.

Table 6 - Impact of Some Stressful Life Events		
Life Event	**Scale of Impact**	
Death of spouse	100	_____
Divorce	73	_____
Martial separation	65	_____
Jail term	63	_____
Death of close family member	63	_____
Personal injury, illness	53	_____
Marriage	50	_____
Fired at work	47	_____
Pregnancy	40	_____
In-law trouble	29	_____
Change in residence	20	_____
Vacation	13	_____

Patients check any life changes they have undergone during the past 2 years, and this is scored against a master scale. A score in the range of 0–150 indicates no significant problems, or low or tolerable levels of life changes. A score of 150–199 indicates mild life changes and is linked to a 33% chance of illness developing. A score of 200–299 indicates moderate life change, or about a 50% chance of illness. When the score is 300 or more, the patient is undergoing major life changes and has an approximately 80% chance of illness developing. Modified forms of the life-stress scale are also available for different ethnic and age groups.

The State-Trait Anxiety Inventory is a similar instrument. It provides 20 items that pertain to the amount of tension or anxiety the patient feels at that moment (state) and 20 items that pertain to the way the patient generally feels (trait). Patients read a general statement and then select a number between 1 and 4 (1 = not at all, 2 = somewhat, 3 = moderately, 4 = very much so) that seems most pertinent to their situation. Sample state statements are

I feel at ease.	(1) (2) (3) (4)
I am worried.	(1) (2) (3) (4)

Sample trait statements are:

I wish I could be as happy as others seem to be.

(1) (2) (3) (4)

I am content.   (1) (2) (3) (4)

The Menninger Clinic and Foundation is a world-famous psychiatric facility in Topeka, Kansas. The Menninger Foundation Biofeedback Center has a stress management seminar in which participants list sources of stress. After they list as many stressors as possible, patients write the number associated with each stressor in a section of a circle that describes the area of life in which the stressor occurs (*Figure 6)*. If it is a stressor that is particularly troublesome, the patient places the number closer to the center of the circle (the center of the circle represents the patient).

These are but a few of the psychological stress indexes that can be used. They may uncover life stresses that may have a real impact on the development of cardiovascular disease.

FAMILY HISTORY

About 5% of families in the general population account for about 50% of early coronary deaths, or deaths from cardiac disease before age 55 (Hopkins et al. 1984). In such high-risk families, first-degree relatives of early coronary victims have a threefold to 10-fold increased risk for early coronary disease. Some families have dominant genes that lead to heart attacks before age 45 in almost all males in their families. Thus, males in the current generation are at increased risk of CHD, and preventive action and follow-up are necessary to prevent coronary disease (Williams et al., 1988).

Other families have a strong predisposition to stroke. This disease could be prevented by effective screening for high blood pressure and appropriate treatment.

As mentioned in earlier chapters, hypercholes-terolemia, cigarette smoking, and hypertension are risk factors that can be modified. They play a major role in most CHD-prone family members.

A thorough history usually uncovers a family history of cardiac problems as well as risk factors for cardiac disease. Many groups, such as the AHA and the American Medical Association, have stressed the importance of uncovering cardiovascular risk as early as possible. Along this line, groups at the University of Utah and Baylor University recently developed a questionnaire that uncovers coronary problems as early as the high school years. The Health Family Tree method devised by Roger Williams, director of the Cardiovascular Genetics Research Clinic at the University of Utah Medical School, and his colleagues, uses a medical family history questionnaire that collects detailed information about disease and risk factors in siblings, parents, aunts, uncles, and grandparents of high school students (Williams et al., 1988). Thirty-seven high schools in 14 communities in Texas and Utah participated in this study. The 24,332 family trees developed from the questionnaire turned up more than 2,666 families at risk of early coronary disease or stroke.

The study showed that many students did not know much of the information asked in the questionnaire but learned about it once they asked their parents. Parents were given 1 week to complete the form by contacting relatives. The students then completed the questionnaires. High-risk families were found to have about 14 asymptomatic high-risk individuals who were first-degree relatives of people who had multiple diseases.

One of the positive results of the program was that teachers, students, and the students' families had a chance to discuss the risks of cardiovascular disease and health strategies to adopt to reduce the risks, such as changing high-fat diets, adding more exercise, and finding ways to reduce or better deal with emotional stresses in everyday life. The researchers also began developing brochures and handouts about reducing the risk for heart disease. This study underscored the importance of using a thorough family history to uncover risk for CHD.

SIGNS AND SYMPTOMS OF CORONARY HEART DISEASE

Not every patient with heart disease has outward signs and symptoms, and not every patient with signs and symptoms of CHD actually has heart disease. A patient may have heart disease without signs and symptoms. Or, signs and symptoms that seem to indicate heart disease may arise from other body systems. Thus, during the history, it is a good idea to ask about all signs and symptoms and to record the patient's response in detail, including the location, radiation, intensity, and duration (Breu, 1987). The signs and symptoms that patients with cardiovascular disease are most likely to report include chest pain; pain in the extremities; dyspnea; palpitations; syncope; near-syncope; dizziness; fatigue; hemoptysis; cyanosis; and edema, particularly edema of the ankles (Chung, 1986).

The focus in this section is on signs and symptoms most often reported that are connected with heart disease. The following general guidelines can be applied to all of them. Questions about each symptom or sign, should include the following (Chung, 1986):

1. The location of the pain, including the area of origin and the duration of the pain.

2. The quality of the pain, that is, a thorough description of the pain—sharp, dull, or boring, for example. Chest pain is often graded on a 10-point scale; for example a 1 signifies pain that is "barely there," whereas chest pain that is intolerable would be rated as 10.

3. The degree, or quantity, of the pain. This includes severity, frequency, and duration. A patient may say, "It is a dull pain that lasts at least 30 min after I eat."

4. The chronology of the pain. This includes onset and development. When did the pain or pains first start, and has pain increased or decreased since the first episode?

5. The setting in which pain occurs. For example, does it occur after meals, during sleep, or in the early morning hours?

6. Factors that aggravate the pain. For example, does the pain occur only after strenuous exercise? Or, is it worsened by stress?

7. Other signs and symptoms that occur with the pain. For example, does the patient have nausea and vomiting as well as pain?

8. Factors that alleviate the pain. For example, lying down alleviates pain.

9. Medication that alleviates the pain. Which medications or methods relieve the pain best?

Chest pain. Chest pain may be due to angina pectoris, MI, pericarditis, myocarditis, pulmonary embolism, dissection of the aorta or mitral valve prolaps; to less serious causes such as psychoneurotic problems, including hyperventilation; or to pneumonia, hiatal hernia, esophageal dysfunction, or gallbladder disease. The characteristics of the major types of cardiac pain are described in the following sections. In most cases, sudden onset of severe chest pain will result in the patient being taken to an emergency department or facility. Less severe pain may be self-diagnosed as "indigestion" or "heartburn" and ignored until it does become severe.

Angina pectoris. Pain from angina pectoris is characterized by paroxysmal attacks of chest discomfort that occur because the coronary blood flow is not sufficient to meet the heart muscle's metabolic demands. Patients may describe the pain as dull and constant, reporting that it seems to be "constricting," "boring," "pressing," or "expanding." It can also be reported as a burning sensation that reminds the patient of "heartburn" or "indigestion." The pain often begins retrosternally and often radiates to the neck, jaws, shoulders, or one or both arms. Often it radiates across the precordium to the left shoulder and upper arm.

The pain can range from mild discomfort to excruciating and occurs at various times. Attacks usually last a few minutes (less than 15), often occur during physical exertion and emotional stress, and are relieved by rest or sublingual nitroglycerin. Angina may also occur during eating, micturition, or defecation and may be affected by cold or by hot, humid weather. When angina occurs increasingly and with ever greater severity, it is termed "unstable angina," or "crescendo angina." When an attack of angina is not relieved by rest and two or more sublingual nitroglycerin tablets, suspect impending acute MI.

Myocardial infarction. The pain of MI differs from angina. First, it is usually more severe and lasts longer. In some cases it can last for hours. When it occurs as a feeling of pressure or a dull, pressing sensation or soreness, it may last from 1 to 3 days. In contrast to angina, it more often occurs during rest and is not relieved by nitroglycerin. It can also occur with emotional or physical exertion. Patients may report having severe pressure or a deep sensation of "crushing," "squeezing," or "indigestion." Other signs and symptoms such as apprehension, nausea, dyspnea, diaphoresis, increased blood pressure, and irregular heart rate may accompany the chest pain associated with an MI.

The pain of an impending MI also usually occurs with a host of other signs and symptoms. For example, the chest pain may be accompanied by life-threatening arrhythmias, which could lead to sudden death.

Pericarditis. The pain of pericarditis is generally sharp, often severe, and usually is located in the precordium; it then radiates into the shoulders and neck. The pain worsens when the patient moves, laughs, coughs, or turns from side to side and is sometimes relieved when the patient leans forward. Because pericarditis can be caused by many disorders, including viral pericarditis, malignant tumors, or tuberculosis, the pain can vary widely.

Patients may describe the pain of pericarditis as "knifelike" or "stabbing" and report it as a mild ache or a severe pain that can be either deep or superficial. It can be precipitated by bacterial, fungal, or viral infection; after cardiac injury, such as MI; trauma; or surgery.

Pulmonary embolism. In contrast to angina, pericarditis, and MI, most small pulmonary emboli produce little or no chest pain. If pain is present with pulmonary emboli, it is usually sharp, starts suddenly, and is aggravated by breathing. Most patients also have marked dyspnea. When pulmonary embolism is suspected, look for a history of recent surgery, pregnancy, trauma, prolonged bed rest, prolonged sitting or standing, or use of oral contraceptives (particularly in smokers).

Psychoneurotic pain. Psychoneurotic pain may be caused by a number of disorders, but anxiety is the most common underlying problem. The pain usually occurs in the inframammary region and rarely radiates. Such pain generally does not occur during physical exertion but may follow such exertion. Often, this pain can be easily linked to other psychological problems, such as severe stress. The hyperventilation syndrome is a good example of a psychological disorder that can cause chest pain.

Pain in the chest wall. Pain in the chest wall is usually due to disorders in the ribs, muscles, xiphoid, nerves, breast, or pleural lining. Fractures, herpes zoster, and a host of disorders can also produce this type of pain. Usually the history will quickly rule out a cardiac-based problem in such patients.

Extremity pain. Pain in the extremities can be due to intermittent claudication or thrombophlebitis. The patient may describe the pain of intermittent claudication as "pins and needles" or "a cramp" or may report that the leg seems to be "going to sleep."

Superficial thrombophlebitis is often marked by pain; erythema; warmth; and a tender, indurated cord running along the vein. Most patients do not have generalized edema. If an older patient has recurrent superficial thrombophlebitis, a search should be made for the possibility of an occult malignant tumor. Deep thrombophlebitis produces pain, swelling, and tenderness in the calf.

Dyspnea. Dyspnea is the distress patients feel when they have difficulty breathing. Dyspnea may result from heart failure, when cardiac output fails to keep pace with increased metabolic needs during activity. As a result, the respiratory drive is increased, largely because of tissue acidosis. The patient's shortness of breath is often accompanied by feelings of lassitude or a feeling of smothering or an oppressive feeling over the sternum. Exertional dyspnea is usually due to congestive heart failure (Chung, 1986). Dyspnea is often triggered by anxiety and hyperventilation.

Orthopnea is a type of dyspnea that occurs when the patient lies down. It usually occurs with left ventricular failure but may also appear with severe pulmonary disease. One clue may be that patients usually use two or more pillows to prop themselves up to sleep. Paroxysmal nocturnal dyspnea is a type of dyspnea that typically occurs 1–2 hr after the patient has fallen asleep.

Palpitations. A palpitation is an uncomfortable or strange feeling in the chest, generally caused by cardiac arrhythmias. The patient will describe the feeling as "my heart is beating too fast," or "beating irregularly," or "skipping beats."

When palpitations are due to premature beats (extrasystoles) or tachyarrhythmias, the patient is often able to describe them in detail, including their frequency, rate, and duration, and can relate them to specific events. Sometimes events other than arrhythmias cause similar sensations of fluttering heartbeat, including vigorous ventricular contractions associated with exercise, anxiety, aortic stenosis, and the hyperkinetic heart syndrome. Murmurs or bruits can also be misinterpreted by the patient as palpitations.

Syncope. Syncope is a transitory loss of consciousness caused by inadequate cerebral blood flow. Near-syncope is light-headedness and weakness without loss of consciousness. The relationship of syncope to activity, palpitations, and body position provides possible clues to its cause. For example, syncope that develops on exertion may be due to aortic stenosis. Syncope that follows palpitations may be caused by an arrhythmia. Syncope that develops when a patient stands up quickly may be due to carotid artery stenosis caused by atherosclerosis, diabetes mellitus, or antihypertensive medication. When turning the head produces syncope, carotid artery stenosis may be the culprit (Chung, 1986). All these possibilities require medical follow-up and substantiated diagnosis.

Fatigue. Fatigue related to cardiovascular disease is usually due to low cardiac output. If volume depletion or potassium depletion occurs, fatigue may follow treatment for heart failure. Patients who are being treated with antihypertensive medications may also feel weakness due to postural hypotension. In addition, ß-blockers used to treat hypertension may cause fatigue, a common side effect of these drugs. The most common cause of fatigue is probably anxiety. Cardiac fatigue is more common with exertion, whereas anxiety-linked fatigue occurs at rest.

Hemoptysis. Hemoptysis can be particularly alarming for patients and dangerous if a large amount of blood is coughed up. Hemoptysis may be caused by the following problems: mitral stenosis, pulmonary infarction, rupture of a pulmonary arteriovenous fistula, rupture of an aortic aneurysm, pulmonary hemosiderosis, or congestive heart failure.

Cyanosis. Cyanosis can be present at birth because of a congenital cardiac anomaly, with left-to-right shunt. It can also be acquired later in life when the patient has congestive heart failure with increases in right-to-left shunt. It may also occur in persons who have severe left ventricular failure. In such cases, the possibility of pulmonary embolism should always be considered.

Thus, a detailed health history is the first step to determining the patient's current state of health and risk of future cardiac disease. The next step in assessment is to use inspection, palpation, auscultation, and percussion to detect physical signs of disease. Steps in a complete physical examination, with emphasis on cardiac evaluation and ways to evaluate physical fitness are covered in the next chapter.

EXAM QUESTIONS

CHAPTER 3
Questions 17–23

17. Which of the following statements about the Health Hazard Appraisal is correct?

    a. Is completed once the results of the physical examination are known.

    b. Uses a questionnaire to develop a computerized profile of patient risk.

    c. Can successfully replace laboratory tests.

    d. Is used for women only.

18. The CAGE questionnaire is helpful for detecting:

    a. Depression

    b. High levels of anxiety

    c. Problems with alcohol

    d. Suicidal tendencies

19. In the Life Change Index, which of the following has the highest impact upon a patient?

    a. Divorce

    b. Being fired

    c. Pregnancy

    d. Death of a spouse

20. About what percentage of families in the general population account for half of early coronary deaths?

    a. 15%

    b. 5%

    c. 25%

    d. 35%

21. True or false: Anginal pain is often described by patients as "boring" or "pressing" and may be mistaken for heartburn or indigestion.

    a. True

    b. False

22. The pain of myocardial infarction (MI) differs from the pain of angina pectoris because the former:

    a. Is usually much more severe and lasts much longer.

    b. Lasts for much shorter periods.

    c. Usually occurs during physical exertion.

    d. Is relieved by nitroglycerin.

23. Fatigue related to cardiovascular disease usually is due to volume depletion.

    a. True

    b. False

CHAPTER 4

ASSESSING PATIENTS FOR CORONARY HEART DISEASE: PHYSICAL EXAMINATION

CHAPTER OBJECTIVE

After studying this chapter, the reader will be able to apply some of the basic principles of physical examination, using inspection, palpation, percussion, and auscultation to detect signs of heart disease.

LEARNING OBJECTIVES

After studying this chapter, the reader should be able to

1. Name three dermatologic signs that may indicate underlying CHD.

2. List at least three guidelines for avoiding errors on blood pressure readings.

3. Describe the four sites where auscultation of the heart is most successful.

4. Explain the difference between a diastolic murmur and a systolic murmur.

INTRODUCTION

After compiling the information from the health history, the nurse can turn to the physical examination. Examining a patient for physical signs of internal disease is as old as medicine itself. Although physical diagnosis has been vastly improved by the development of modern testing devices, many of the clues to unde-

tected CHD can be found by using the time-honored methods of inspection, palpation, percussion, and auscultation.

This chapter concentrates on these four methods of examining patients and on physical fitness tests the nurse can use to uncover or verify the presence of or increased risk of CHD developing. Later chapters focus on individual testing methods, including resting and stress electrocardiography (ECG), echocardiography, angiography, and nuclear medicine tests.

GENERAL SCREENING TESTS

The timing and frequency of regular medical examinations is still a controversial issue. Some advocate annual physical examinations for all adults. Others think that routine screening of the general population is expensive and not very efficient, because the cost does not seem to justify the information gained. The debate also extends to regular screening for cardiovascular risk. The AHA (1987) takes the position that prevention is the greatest need for cardiovascular health and has stated that many cardiovascular diseases, especially atherosclerotic disease, can be prevented by regular examinations to detect risk factors for CHD.

How often should the average asymptomatic person have a general physical examination? The AHA has stated that apparently healthy people between 20 and 60 years of age should have routine examinations at least once every 5 years, beginning at age 20. At the first evaluation, a medical history should be taken, a physical examination done, and baseline information recorded. At each visit, the blood pressure should be measured, the subject weighed; and fasting levels of plasma cholesterol, triglycerides, and glucose measured. A baseline resting ECG should also be obtained at age 20, then repeated at ages 40 and 60 in normotensive patients. Blood pressure should be measured once at the midpoint between the 5-year examinations. A baseline chest film should be taken at age 40. Those who are older than 60 should be examined at least every 2.5 years until they reach 75. During these visits, it is often a good idea to measure levels of plasma lipids, although this is optional. After age 75, patients should be examined once a year. Then, with each subsequent visit, the data from the previous examination should be updated.

The AHA recommends the following to evaluate the cardiovascular system during a routine physical examination:

1. Examination of rate, rhythm, and contour of arterial and venous pulses.

2. Measurement of blood pressure in both arms with the patient supine or seated, then standing.

3. Examination for carotid bruits.

4. Ocular examination, searching for corneal arcus and changes in the fundus, including arteriovenous compression, hemorrhages, exudates, and papilledema.

5. Heart rate, rhythm, apex impulse, other precordial impulses, heart murmurs, third or fourth heart sounds or gallops, ejection or nonejection clicks.

6. Examination of the chest for shape, motion on respiration, presence of rales, and transmitted heart murmurs.

7. Examination of the abdomen for bruits, enlarged kidneys or other organs, and dilatation of the aorta.

8. Examination of the extremities for diminution or absence of peripheral arterial pulsations, edema, clubbing, and varicose veins.

9. Examination of the nervous system.

STANDARD MEASUREMENTS

Physical examination often begins with standard measurements, such as weight and height. Height is measured while the patient is in his or her stocking feet. Weight is measured with the patient wearing lightweight clothing. Many patients volunteer to get rid of coats and other heavy clothing to try to save a pound or two on the scale.

Body weight and body fat. The most commonly used measurement for the relative, or desirable, weight is the standard tables based on height and sex. The Metropolitan Life Insurance Company's weight tables are perhaps the most widely used (Metropolitan Life Insurance Company, 1983). Such tables define desirable weight as the weight that has been associated with the lowest mortality rates among people buying life insurance. Such tables generally divide desirable weights into three types of body frame: large, medium, and small. A range of desirable weights is listed for each height and frame category.

Determining the percentage of body fat is another way to measure weight and body fat. With this method, a skinfold caliper is used to measure body density and to calculate the percentage of body fat and lean tissue. A skinfold (defined as two layers of skin and subcutaneous fat, not muscle) on

Table 7
Guidelines for Girth Measurements

WOMEN

Bust and hips: same

Abdomen (measured at waist): 25–26 cm less than bust and hips

Thigh: 15 cm less than waist

Calf: 15–18 cm less than thigh

Ankle: 13–15 cm less than calf

Biceps, relaxed: twice the size of the wrist

MEN

Chest and hips: same

Abdomen at waist: 20–25 cm less than chest and hips

Thigh: 20–25 cm less than abdomen

Calf: 18–20 cm less than thigh

Ankle: 15–18 cm less than calf

Biceps, relaxed: twice the size of the wrist

the right side of the body is grasped with one hand, and the skinfold caliper is applied about 1 cm below the skinfold. Skinfolds are picked up in the vertical plane, except for the subscapular and suprailiac areas, where the skin is grasped at a slight angle. Skinfold measurements are made at four sites: the triceps, subscapular area, suprailiac region, and outer thigh. Each skinfold should be measured three times by regrasping the fold; then, the average value of the two closest measurements is used as the final measurement (Pender, 1987).

The next step in calculating the percentage of body fat is to calculate the body density. The following are the formulas for men and women (Getchell, 1980):

Men: Body density (g/cm³) = 1.1043 - $(0.00131 \times$ subscapula measurement [mm] - $(0.001327 \times$ thigh measurement [mm])

Women: Body density (g/cm³) = 1.0764 -

$(0.00088 \times$ triceps measurement [mm])
$(0.00081 \times$ suprailiac measurement [mm])

The percentage of body fat is then computed by the following formula:

Percentage of body fat = (4.570/body density − 4.142) × 100

Lean body weight can be calculated with the following formula:

Fat weight = body weight (kg) × % body fat × 100

Lean body weight = body weight - fat weight

For men, desirable weight should equal lean weight/0.88 (12% body fat). For women, desired weight should equal lean weight/0.82 (18% of body fat).

Girth measurements. Although there are as many variations on normal as there are individual patients, some rough guidelines for appropriate body proportions have been established by exercise physiologists such as Leroy Getchell, director of physical fitness programs at The Human Performance Laboratory at Ball State University, Muncie, Indiana. Normal proportions for men and women are shown in *Table 7.*

This is also a good point at which to evaluate the patient's nutrition. Current dietary patterns and the percentage of types of nutrients should also be assessed. One helpful tool is to have a patient keep a record of all food and drink consumed for 5–7 days before the physical examination or before the first visit. The record can be kept on a food diary form that shows the types of food and drink and amounts consumed during regular meals and snacks. Once the nurse has the food diary, computerized programs and charts are available to convert the food intake for each day to glucose, protein, and carbohydrates (Suitor & Hunter, 1980). The nurse can also work with the patient to change harmful eating patterns, for example, to reduce daily percentages of saturated fats and refined and processed sugars. A later chapter presents some programs and approaches that can be used to help improve overall nutrition.

Results of some laboratory studies will also help determine nutritional status. Some helpful tests include levels of blood urea nitrogen, cholesterol, serum protein, and serum albumin; plasma vitamin levels; and plasma calcium, potassium, iron, phosphorus, and magnesium levels.

Blood pressure. Normal blood pressure is defined as a diastolic blood pressure less than 85 mm Hg and a systolic blood pressure less than 130 mm Hg. When diastolic blood pressure falls between 85 and 89 mm Hg, it is called "high-normal." Such patients are thought to be at higher than normal risk for cardiovascular disease.

Diastolic and systolic blood pressure readings should be obtained on three separate occasions when establishing a baseline value, because a number of factors, such as stress or anxiety, can increase or decrease blood pressure. To avoid falsely increased blood pressure, the AHA recommends that blood pressure not be measured immediately after a stressful or physically taxing situation (Kirkendall et al., 1980).

Before the blood pressure is measured, the patient should sit quietly for at least 5 min and should wait at least 30 min after drinking coffee or tea, eating, or smoking. The patient should be seated comfortably, with the arm positioned properly. Watch that a rolled up sleeve does not constrict the upper arm. The diastolic pressure is the last sound heard as the arm cuff is deflated. Remember to use a large-sized cuff for obese patients. Other suggestions are to have the sphygmomanometer regularly calibrated and to measure blood pressure in both arms. Also remember that there may be "skip" areas, the so-called auscultatory gap, where interruptions in the Korotkoff

sounds are heard in hypertensive patients. Blood pressure readings should be taken with the patient first lying down and then standing up. A difference of more than 15 mm Hg between the two readings may be a sign of poorly controlled hypertension, aortic disease, or cerebrovascular disease (Miracle, 1988).

The pulse pressure, or the difference between systolic and diastolic pressures, should also be determined. A pulse pressure greater than 40 mm Hg may suggest a condition that leads to enlarged ventricles, aortic regurgitation, or coronary artery disease. A pulse pressure less than 30 mm Hg may indicate a condition that results from reduced cardiac output, such as aortic stenosis or heart failure.

Table 8 gives the suggested follow-up for patients found to have elevated diastolic and systolic measurements on regular examinations.

After hypertension is diagnosed, a search for the underlying cause should begin. Some people with mild hypertension may respond to nonpharmacologic treatment, such as reducing sodium in the diet or a reducing diet. In many obese people, blood pressure returns to normal as excess weight is lost. In some people, drinking more than 2 oz (60 ml) of alcohol or its equivalent daily raises blood pressure. Also, certain routinely prescribed and over-the-counter medications can raise blood pressure. Here are a few drugs that can raise blood pressure: oral contraceptives, nose drops, postmenopausal estrogens, other steroids, nonsteroidal antiinflammatory drugs, and antacids containing sodium.

Always look for secondary causes for elevated blood pressure. The medical history may reveal the cause, such as Cushing disease or renal disease. Laboratory tests that may help pinpoint the cause include hemoglobin and hematocrit, complete urinalysis, serum potassium, and serum creatinine.

Table 8
Recommendations for Follow-up for Adults Based on Initial Set of Blood Pressure Measurements

Initial Screening Blood Pressure, mm Hg*		
Systolic	**Diastolic**	**Follow-up Recommended†**
<130	<85	Recheck in 2 y
130–139	85–89	Recheck in 1 y‡
140–159	90–99	Confirm within 2 mo
160–179	100–109	Evaluate or refer to source of care within 1 mo
180–209	110–119	Evaluate or refer to source of care within 1 wk
≥210	≥120	Evaluate or refer to source of care immediately

* *If the systolic and diastolic categories are different, follow recommendation for the shorter-time follow-up (eg. 160/85 mm Hg should be evaluated or referred to source of care within 1 month).*
† *The scheduling of follow-up should be modified by reliable information about past blood pressure measurements, other cardiovascular risk factors, or target-organ disease.*
‡ *Consider providing advice about life-style modifications.*

Reprinted with permission from: The fifth report of the Joint National Committee on Detection, Evaluation & Treatment of High Blood Pressure (1993). *Archives of Internal Medicine, 153,* 163.

INSPECTION

You can learn a lot about patients by carefully observing them. First, is the patient calm, anxious, tired, or full of energy? Does the patient show any distress? Is the patient gaunt or obese? As noted before, obesity is one of the most common risk factors for development of cardiovascular disease, including angina pectoris and MI.

Changes in the skin. Search for and ask about any skin changes, particularly those that may be related to poor circulation, such as brittle hair; dry, shiny skin; and thickened nails, especially toenails (Breu, 1987). The patient's general skin color can also provide clues to possible cardiovascular disease. Cyanosis is a major sign, which might indicate congenital heart anomaly, congestive heart failure, or a number of types of vascular disease. Cyanosis is not always a danger sign, however. There are two types of cyanosis to keep in mind. Peripheral cyanosis can be seen in patients who are cold or anxious and is found on the fingertips and lips. This occurs in exposed parts of the body and disappears with warming. Central cyanosis, however, which causes blueness around the mouth and lips, as well as in the nail beds, is a sign of major oxygenation deficiency, usually caused by heart or lung disease. Generalized cyanosis may also be due to underlying anemia.

Generalized pallor or discoloration of the skin may indicate impaired cardiac output or underlying anemia from a number of causes. For example, it may result from decreasing levels of oxygenated hemoglobin. Localized pallor or trophic lesions suggest impaired regional blood flow. Generalized pallor is often hard to evaluate because of the many differences and varieties of normal skin tones. Because of this variation, pallor is detected in the patient's conjunctiva, mouth and nails.

The opposite condition, generalized flushing of the skin, may be caused by peripheral vasodilation, a sign of increased cardiac output. You may detect this in patients who are pregnant or who have thy-

Figure 7
Inspection of External Jugular Venous Pressure

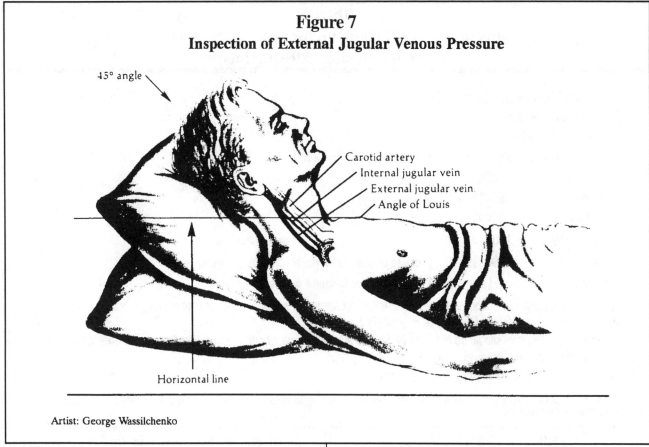

45° angle

Carotid artery
Internal jugular vein
External jugular vein
Angle of Louis

Horizontal line

Artist: George Wassilchenko

rotoxicosis or arteriovenous fistulas. Jaundice occurs with late congestive heart failure and is easiest to see in the sclerae of the eye under natural light.

Clubbing of the nails. Clubbing of the nails is common in people with lung cancer, chronic obstructive lung disease, and congenital cardiovascular disease. With clubbing, the angle between the nail fold and the nail bed disappears. Some patients have normal, familial rounding of the nails, and this can be differentiated from true clubbing by examining the angle between the nail bed and the finger. Normally, this angle is 160°. With clubbing, the angle is greater than 160°. Clubbing can also cause abnormal convexity of the nails and widening and thickening of the terminal phalanges of both the hands and the feet. To detect this, look at the depth of the distal phalanges and the depth of the interphalanges. With clubbing, the distal phalangeal depth is greater.

Jugular venous pulse. Venous distension or abnormal pulses in the neck may indicate right-sided heart failure, right-sided valvular disease, or cardiac tamponade. To evaluate this, place the patient at a 45° angle, so that the internal jugular vein can be observed. Make sure that the patient's head is not turned enough to tense the tissues of the neck, which will obscure the pulse wave (Chung, 1986 *Figure 7*).

The best area to view the pulses is on either side of the neck. The reference point is the angle at which the manubrium joins the sternum. Arterial and venous pulses can be differentiated by the following characteristics (Chung, 1986):

1. The venous pulse can not be palpated.

2. The venous pulse normally has three distinct waves, rather than the single wave of the arterial pulse.

3. Venous pulsations and distension normally decrease when the patient sits up after being in a reclining position.

4. Inspiration decreases venous pulsations and distension by increasing the filling of the right side of the heart. The Valsalva maneuver produces the opposite effect.

You can then observe the internal jugular vein to find the highest level of visible pulsation. Next, find the sternal notch by palpating the clavicles at the point where they join the sternum. Place the first two fingers on the suprasternal notch, then, keeping them on the skin, slide them down the sternum until the bony prominence is found, the angle of Louis (Breu, 1987). Then, the venous pressure can be estimated by measuring the vertical distance between the highest level of visible pulsation and the angle of Louis. This is normally less than 3 cm. Add 5 cm to the measurement, to estimate the total distance between the highest level of pulsation and the right atrium. If the total is more than 10 cm, the patient may have elevated venous pressure; suspect right-sided heart failure.

Venous pressure can be estimated by using the veins of the hand or the internal or external jugular veins. When examining the veins of the hand, the patient should lie at about a 30° angle. The hand should be held below the level of the heart until the veins fill and then should be gradually lifted until the veins collapse. This usually happens at about the level of the sternal angle on the chest (Chung, 1986).

If the external jugular veins of the neck are used, the trunk should be elevated 30° to 60°. Compress the vein lightly by placing a finger just superior and parallel to the clavicle. After the vein has filled, compression can be withdrawn, and the angle of filling above the sternal angle can be observed. It is normally less than 3 cm. If the internal jugular vein is used to estimate venous pressure, the patient is positioned at the same position, and the vertical distance above the sternal angle is recorded. This is also normally less than 3 cm.

What causes elevated venous pressure? The most common cause of elevated venous pressure is right-sided heart failure (Chung, 1986). The Valsalva maneuver can also elevate pressure in the neck veins. Thus, the patient should breathe quietly during the examination of the venous pulse.

After this, a general inspection of the anterior chest, with a systemic approach, to note any apparent abnormalities can be made. Be sure to look at five areas: (a) the aortic area, including the second intercostal space to the right of the sternum; (b) the pulmonic area, the second intercostal space to the left of the sternum; (c) the right ventricular area, the lower half of the left sternal border; (d) the apical area, which is the fifth intercostal space along the midclavicular line; and (e) the epigastric area, near the xiphoid process.

PALPATION

Palpating the skin and assessing all peripheral pulses may uncover more clues to underlying cardiovascular problems. This skill requires practice but can easily be learned.

First, feel the patient's skin, checking for general temperature and moisture. Check the skin turgor by gently lifting a fold of the skin, then seeing how quickly it returns to its former position. If the skin sluggishly returns to normal, the patient may have dehydration. Then, check for signs of edema, especially in the legs, sacrum, and lower legs. When swollen areas are found, press them with one or more fingers to see if indurations result (pitting edema) (Breu, 1987).

Check all peripheral pulses, including the carotids, brachials, radials, femorals, popliteals, dorsalis pedis, and posterial tibials, and record their rate, quality, and equality. These pulses should be bilaterally equal. All pulses should be rated on a scale of 0 to 4+. (*Table 9* shows normal values for peripheral pulses.) Normally, the peripheral pulses arrive later, have a steeper rise and fall, and are generally less helpful than the carotid pulse for providing information about ventricular ejection. Also, be sure to monitor the radial pulse for 1 full min, noting its rhythm, regularity, or irregularity. It can be graded on the same 0 to 4 scale: 0 = absent; 1 = decreased or diminished; 2 = normal; 3 = full or increased; and 4 = bounding.

Arterial pulses. Palpating the arterial pulses will enable you to determine the heart rate and underlying cardiac rhythm, as well as any extra beats. It will also help to determine the patency of the arteries and the characteristics of the pulse waves.

The patient should be placed in a reclining position at about a 30° to 45° angle with the head turned just slightly toward the ipsilateral (or same) side. Apply just enough pressure with a fingertip to feel the arterial waveform. Then, measure the arterial pulse rate and auscultate the heart rate at the same time, to draw a comparison.

While checking the arterial pulses, you may discover an alteration in the pulse, in which weak impulses alternate with strong impulses (pulsus alternans). If you suspect pulsus alternans, apply a blood pressure cuff and raise the pressure above the systolic level. Gradually lower the pressure. In the beginning, you will hear only stronger beats. Then, the pulse rate will double as the pressure is lowered, and you will be able to hear the weaker beats as well. This may be a sign of ventricular failure.

Paradoxical pulse, or pulsus paradoxus, is another abnormal sign that may be detected during

Table 9
Normal Values for the Peripheral Pulses

Pulse	Right	Left
Temporal	2+	2+
Carotid	3+	3+
Brachial	2+	2+
Femoral	2+	2+
Popliteal	2+	2+
Posterior tibialis	2+	2+
Dorsalis pedis	2+	2+

Source: Breu, C. S. (1987). Assessment: Review of vital skills. In *Combating cardiovascular diseases skillfully.* Springhouse, PA: Springhouse Publishing Company.

palpation. Normally, when a patient inspires, the systolic blood pressure falls about 4–8 mm Hg. With pulsus paradoxus, the pressure falls more than 10 mm Hg. The way to detect paradoxical pulse is to apply a blood pressure cuff and raise the pressure to the systolic level so that beats can be heard when the patient expires. Slowly deflate the cuff until you hear impulses when the patient inspires and expires. The difference between the first and second reading is the paradoxical pulse. It may be a sign of underlying constrictive pericarditis, cardiac tamponade, emphysema, or bronchial asthma (Chung, 1986). Record the size of the carotid, radial, brachial, femoral, popliteal, dorsalis pedis, and posterior tibial pulses and compare them with the contralateral (or opposite) pulse.

After doing this, palpate the chest systematically, just as it was inspected. Carefully feel the aortic, pulmonic, right ventricular, apical, and epigastric areas, feeling for pulsations or thrills (vibrations that will remind you of a cat's purr).

In the apical area, look for the apical impulse, which is usually found in the fifth intercostal space at the left midclavicular line. This is the point of maximal impulse, or PMI, and correlates with ventricular systole. It will provide information about abnormalities of the left ventricle. The PMI is generally about 2 cm in diameter, begins with the first heart sound, and lasts only until the middle of systole. When the PMI is larger than normal or found more laterally than normal, it could indicate that the patient has left-sided valvular disease, coronary artery disease, or hypertension. If it is forceful and lasts longer than usual, the patient may have left ventricular hypertrophy. Left ventricular gallops may also be found in this general area: You will feel a lift in the left parasternal area during systole (Breu, 1987).

PERCUSSION

The value of percussion is still being debated, and this technique is rarely included in a standard cardiovascular examination. Some think that it contributes little to the cardiovascular workup, whereas others note that it can be useful for showing abnormally increased dullness to the right of the sternum (Chung, 1986). This may be caused by dextrocardia, loss of volume of the right lung with mediastinal displacement, tension pneumothorax of the left lung, or large pericardial effusions.

One use for percussion is to help estimate heart size, although the standard chest radiograph is a more accurate technique. Usually the patient lies supine. It is best to begin at the fifth intercostal space and move to the fourth if needed. Percuss toward the sternum until dullness is heard. This point of dullness, or change in the note, is the left border of cardiac dullness. In an average adult male, this point is usually 10–12 cm from the midsternal line, always within the midclavicular line. The heart may be enlarged if the left border of cardiac dullness is farther than 12 cm from the midsterum and outside the midclavicular line. This can be a normal finding when the patient is a well-trained athlete (Breu, 1987).

If any abnormalities have been detected during inspection, palpation, and percussion, it may be possible to confirm them with a third step, auscultation. An explanation for this procedure follows.

AUSCULTATION

A few factors that will improve the accuracy of auscultation include an examining room free of extraneous noises; a relaxed and comfortable patient; and a stethoscope equipped with a bell (to hear low-pitched sounds), a diaphragm (to hear higher pitched sounds), and well-fitting earpieces. It may be necessary to have the patient assume several different positions, including sitting, lying down, and lying in the left lateral position. In addition, having the patient perform several different maneuvers, such as Valsalva's maneuver, squatting, and quickly standing up, may help you assess suspected murmurs.

The key to successful auscultation is to focus on one heart sound at a time. It is also helpful to review the hemodynamics of the cardiac cycle. You can easily link each element of the cardiac cycle to the sounds heard, for example, the opening and closing of each of the heart valves and the points at which systole and diastole occur. When using the diaphragm, you should apply it to the chest with relatively heavy pressure (Chung, 1986). Low-frequency sounds such as gallop rhythms and mitral and tricuspid stenosis murmurs are best heard with the bell of the stethoscope. The bell is an effective tool when it is placed lightly on the chest wall, with just enough pressure to form an airtight seal with the skin.

The first step is to determine the patient's heart rate and rhythm. A discrepancy between the apical heart rate and the peripheral pulse rate indicates less effective peripheral perfusion with some heart beats, or a pulse deficit.

Events in each heart valve are best heard at four main areas over the precordium. Sounds related to motion of each heart valve are reflected to a specific area of the chest wall. These locations are not necessarily related to the anatomic position of the valve, nor do all sounds in the area originate in the valve that names it (Chung, 1986). The four

Figure 8

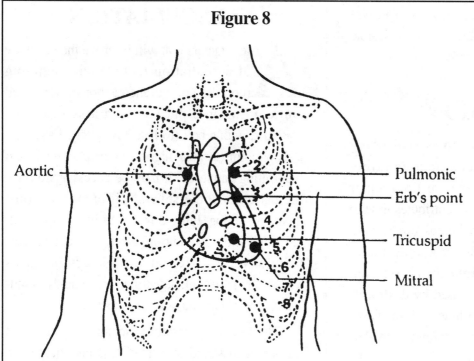

Auscultation sites. The second intercostal space at the right sternal border is referred to as the aortic area; the second intercostal space at the left sternal border is referred to as the pulmonic area; the third intercostal space at the left sternal border is Erb's point; the fifth intercostal space at the left sternal border is referred to as the tricuspid area or lower left sternal border; the fifth intercostal space at midclavicular line is referred to as the mitral area or apical area.

Source: Holloway, N. M., *Nursing the critically ill adult,* 3rd. ed., Addison-Wesley Co., Menlo Park, 1988.

Finally, the tricuspid area, the fourth and fifth interspaces to the left of the sternum, is a good place to detect murmurs of tricuspid stenosis, insufficiency, and ventricular septal defects. Murmurs caused by aortic insufficiency are also heard well in this area.

You have to be sure that you have thoroughly listened to the heart sounds, it is best to use a systematic approach, starting at the aortic area and slowly working to each of the other valve areas. Some suggest going through the four sites with the diaphragm and then using the bell over the same sites (Breu, 1987).

areas are: (a) the cardiac apex, (b) the pulmonic area, (c) the aortic area, and (d) the tricuspid area *(Figure 8)*.

The cardiac apex is the best spot to listen for mitral valve murmurs, the opening snap that signals mitral stenosis, and nonejection clicks. Gallop sounds and rubs can be heard very well in this area.

The pulmonic area, the second and third left intercostal spaces (the third left intercostal space is also called Erb's point) close to the sternum, is a good site to listen for murmurs originating in the pulmonic valve. The pulmonic part of the second heart sound and the murmur of patent ductus arteriosus can also be heard.

The aortic area, the second intercostal space to the right of the sternum, is a good region to listen for murmurs originating at the aortic junction. Aortic ejection clicks also commonly are heard in this region.

The four heart sounds. The four heart sounds, S_1 through S_4, allow you to trace the cardiac cycle as each of the heart valves closes.

The first heart sound, S_1, occurs at the beginning of ventricular systole and is associated with closure of the mitral and tricuspid valves. Pressure rises in the ventricles until it becomes higher than atrial pressure. The atrioventricular valves thus are forced to close. As they close, the first heart sound is transmitted to the chest wall. Normally it is loudest at the apex of the heart, and the mitral valve closes slightly before the tricuspid valve, so that an audible splitting of the first heart sound is common and normal. These two sounds occur 0.2–0.3 sec apart.

Listen for intensity, consistency, and splitting.

The second heart sound, S_2, is associated with closure of the aortic and pulmonic valves. As systole ends and the ventricle begins to relax, a slight backflow of blood in the pulmonary artery and in the aorta occurs, and this causes the pulmonic and aortic valves to close. The sound transmitted to the chest wall is the second heart sound. Because it is associated with closure of both of these valves, it is loudest at Erb's point or can be heard at the base (upper area) of the heart.

Normally, the aortic valve closes first, followed by closure of the pulmonic valve, but the interval is so short between the two that S_2 often seems like a single sound. Abnormally wide splitting of the second heart sound occurs with conditions that cause delayed pulmonary valve closure or early aortic valve closure, such as right bundle branch block, pulmonic stenosis, and left-to-right shunts (Chung, 1986). Reversed, or paradoxical, splitting of S_2 occurs when aortic closure is delayed to a degree that it is preceded by closure of the pulmonary valve. This may occur with left bundle branch block, aortic stenosis, and left ventricular dysfunction caused by ischemia or cardiomyopathy.

The third heart sound, S_3, occurs during the resting phase of the ventricles, or diastole. The third heart sound is best heard with the bell of the stethoscope as the patient lies in the left lateral position. At the beginning of diastole, the pressure in the atria exceeds the pressure in the ventricles and causes the mitral and tricuspid valves to open. This leads to rapid filling of the ventricles as the blood in the atria rushes into the ventricles. As it courses in, a low-frequency vibration occurs. This is considered normal in children and young adults less than 30 years old. It can also be heard in abnormal conditions such as valvular regurgitation or ventricular failure. S_3 is also called a "diastolic filling sound" or "ventricular gallop."

When left ventricular failure or aortic or mitral valve regurgitation is present, it is best heard over the mitral area. If right ventricular failure or right-sided valvular regurgitation is present, the third

sound is best heard in the tricuspid area. Because an S_3 occurs at the beginning of diastole and a split S_2 occurs at the end of systole, it is necessary to listen carefully at different places to distinguish between S_2 and S_3.

The fourth heart sound, or S_4, occurs as ventricular filling continues throughout diastole and ends with atrial contraction. This is a slow-filling phase that creates the low-frequency sound of S_4. Because it is a low-frequency sound, you can hear it best with the bell of the stethoscope, with the patient lying on his or her left side. An S_4 is often found in patients who have decreased ventricular compliance, such as those with hypertension, semilunar valvular stenosis, coronary artery disease, or an acute MI, and it is often audible in older people (especially those over 65) and is a normal variant.

When the patient has left-sided dysfunction, you can hear S_4 best in the mitral area. When it is due to right-sided dysfunction, you can hear the sound best in the tricuspid area. Because the fourth heart sound appears at the end of diastole and a split first heart sound occurs at the beginning of systole, it is necessary to listen carefully to differentiate the location, pitch, timing, and duration of these sounds.

Murmurs. A heart murmur is the sound of blood flowing through an abnormal opening, such as damaged valves or narrowed or stenosed or poorly closing valves, which allow blood to flow back up through the valve. A murmur might also be described as a series of vibrations that occur when blood velocity becomes critically high across an area of vascular narrowing or when irregularity is present (Breu, 1987). A heart murmur also occurs when a large volume of blood flows through a normal-sized valve opening. Heart murmurs are classified according to timing, intensity, pitch, location, quality, and radiation.

When you are attempting to time a murmur, it is important to establish whether it occurs during diastole, systole, or both. If a murmur is heard with or after the first heart sound and ends at or before the second heart sound, it is a systolic murmur. If it occurs between S_2 and the next S_1, it is a diastolic murmur. Early systolic murmurs begin with the first heart sound and end before the second heart sound occurs and may be caused by acute mitral insufficiency or ventricular septal defect. Late systolic murmurs begin well after the beginning of ventricular ejection and continue to or through the second heart sound. The usual causes are mitral valve prolapse and papillary muscle dysfunction.

The intensity of murmurs is graded from I to VI. A grade I murmur is very faint, and may be missed by inexperienced persons. Grade II is soft and low. Grade III is prominent but not palpable. Grade IV is prominent and palpable (a vibration, or thrill, can be felt). Grade V can be heard with a stethoscope held 1 in. (2.5 cm) from the chest wall. Grade VI is loud enough to be heard without a stethoscope.

Murmurs are also classified by their pitch. A murmur may be low-, medium-, or high-pitched, depending on the velocity of blood flow. To evaluate its pitch, listen to a murmur with both the bell and the diaphragm. If it is heard best with the bell, it is a low-pitched murmur. If it is heard best with the diaphragm, it is a high-pitched murmur. If the sound is heard it equally well with the bell and the diaphragm, it is a medium-pitched murmur.

Murmurs are also classified by place and duration. Murmurs that occur during systole and that are due to left-sided cardiac disease are murmurs of aortic stenosis and mitral regurgitation. Those that occur during systole, because of right-sided disease, are murmurs of pulmonic stenosis and tricuspid regurgitation. Those that occur during diastole, during the time when the left ventricle is filling, are murmurs of tricuspid stenosis and pulmonic regurgitation. Holosystolic murmurs are the result of blood flow from an area of high pressure to one of

lower pressure during the entire systolic cycle.

Here is a summary of types of murmurs:

- A pansystolic or holosystolic murmur lasts during the entire systolic phase.

- An early systolic murmur or ejection murmur starts right after the first heart sound and ends at midsystole.

- A late systolic murmur starts at midsystole and ends at the second heart sound.

- An early diastolic murmur starts with the second heart sound and ends at middiastole.

- A middiastolic murmur starts after the second heart sound and ends before the first heart sound.

- A late diastolic, or presystolic, murmur starts at middiastole and ends at the first heart sound.

- Murmurs that can be heard throughout systole and diastole are termed continuous murmurs.

The quality of a murmur refers to its characteristic pattern and sound. There are four general patterns (Miracle, 1988): (a) A crescendo murmur starts rather softly and builds in intensity. It may be described as "coarse," "rumbling," or "whooping." (b) A decrescendo murmur starts loudly, then lessens in intensity. It may be described as a blowing or whistling sound. (c) A crescendo-decrescendo murmur starts slowly, becomes louder, then softer. It may be described as a harsh, grating, or coarse sound. (d) A plateau murmur sounds the same throughout its duration.

Finally, a murmur can be defined by its pattern of radiation. Usually, the higher the pitch and the greater the intensity, the more likely it is that a murmur will radiate. Knowing where it radiates will help you determine the type of murmur. For example, a murmur due to mitral insufficiency often radiates from the mitral valve to the left axilla.

Many murmurs are classified as benign, innocent, physiologic, or functional. All these terms signify that the murmur is not caused by any cardiovascular disease. Benign murmurs are often heard in children and in pregnant women (Miracle, 1988).

Clicks. Clicks are heart sounds that differ from murmurs in several ways. Most murmurs are sustained, whereas clicks are not. Clicks are short, high-pitched sounds that can occur during systole and diastole and can be best heard with the diaphragm of the stethoscope. There are three general types of clicks: one type, merely called a click; a second type, an ejection sound; and a third type, called the opening click. The first type is heard during systole and is usually due to mitral valve prolapse. The click usually occurs in midsystole, as the valve starts to snap back into the left atrium. It is best heard by using the diaphragm to listen at the left mitral valve area. The ejection sound is caused by ejection of blood from the right ventricle through a defective pulmonic valve or from the left ventricle through a defective aortic valve. The sound is short and high-pitched and occurs early in systole, right after the first heart sound. It is best heard with the diaphragm. The opening click is the sound of the opening of a stenotic mitral valve. Like the other types, it is short in duration and high-pitched. It is best heard by placing the diaphragm between the tricuspid valve area and the mitral valve area. Possible causes include pulmonary embolism or pulmonic stenosis.

Pericardial friction rub. Just like murmurs, pericardial friction rubs are sustained sounds. And, like clicks, they are usually high-pitched. The difference between murmurs and clicks and a pericardial friction rub is the nature of the sound itself. Friction rubs can be described as coarse or scratchy (similar to leather rubbing against leather).

Friction rubs are caused by abnormal movement of the parietal and visceral layers of the pericardial sac. Normally, movement is smooth and silent. However, infection, uremia, or an MI can cause an inflammation (pericarditis). Pericarditis

causes a scratchy sound as the parietal and visceral surfaces rub against each other. Typically, such patients will report precordial chest discomfort, shortness of breath, fever, chills, and weakness.

ASSESSING PHYSICAL FITNESS

You can get a good idea of the patient's general level of activity through the history and by physical examination and laboratory tests. In general, questions about exercise should be directed toward activities that are vigorous or of high intensity (Grundy et al., 1987). **A hint:** The amount of exercise associated with reduced risk of cardiovascular disease is estimated to be 4 or 5 hr a week at a high enough intensity to cause breathlessness.

The hallmark of exercise conditioning is the lowering of the heart rate at rest. Another physiologic indicator of exercise conditioning is the maximal amount of physical work that can be performed during an exercise tolerance test (Grundy et al., 1987). One simple test, the step test, can be done right in the office. A variation of this can be done at home, at the patient's convenience. The step test is a simple version of the stress test. Although it is not as physiologically stressful as the laboratory stress test. It is a good idea to have a physician available for emergency backup if the patient is more than 40 years old, is obese, or has a history of heart problems (Pender, 1987).

Muscle strength and endurance can also be tested by having patients do certain exercises, such as bent knee sit-ups. Flexibility can be judged by the simple action of having them bend over to touch their toes.

When doing bent-knee sit-ups, the patient lies on his or her back, with both knees bent, and sits up while the examiner holds the patient's ankles. For women, the examiner counts the number of sit-ups per minute. For men, the number of sit-ups in 2 min is counted. Older persons or those with cardiovascular problems must be watched carefully for any signs of fatigue, and sit-ups should be immediately stopped if the patient has any signs of distress.

For women, the number of sit-ups in 1 min can signify levels of fitness: 33 or more is excellent, 27–32 is good, 20–26 is average, 16–21 is fair, and 16 or fewer is poor. For men, the scoring is as follows: 69 or more within 2 min is excellent, 60–68

is good, 59–52 is average, 51–42 is fair, and 41 or fewer is poor.

Using inspection, palpation, percussion, and auscultation, with the results of a number of laboratory tests, you can assess the patient's general overall health and risk of CHD. For a number of patients, the results of the history and physical examination will call for a more thorough examination of the heart, as with an ECG. The next chapter focuses on both resting and stress ECGs.

EXAM QUESTIONS

CHAPTER 4

Questions 24–38

24. According to the AHA, how often should apparently healthy people 20–60 years old have a routine physical examination?

    a. Once every 5 years

    b. Once every 3 years

    c. Annually

    d. Only when specific signs andsymptoms occur

25. "High-normal" blood pressure is defined as:

    a. Diastolic pressure 80–85 mm Hg

    b. Diastolic pressure greater than 90 mm Hg

    c. Diastolic pressure 85–89 mm Hg

    d. Diastolic pressure greater than 105 mm Hg

26. What is the generally recommended follow-up for a patient with diastolic pressure between 85 and 89 mm Hg?

    a. Reconfirm within 2 months.

    b. Recheck within 1 year.

    c. Confirm within 2 weeks, and start therapy soon after.

    d. Recheck every 2–3 years.

27. A grade III murmur would best be described as:

    a. Prominent, but not palpable

    b. Loud and palpable

    c. Barely available

    d. Life threatening

28. Which of the following statements about "clubbing" of the nailsis correct?

    a. It creates a flattening of the angle between the nail fold and nail bed.

    b. It creates a narrower distal phalangeal depth.

    c. It is diagnostic of coronary artery disease.

    d. It occurs only in adults.

29. True or false: Cyanosis may be a sign of a serious underlying cardiac problem.

    a. True

    b. False

30. The most common cause of elevated central venous pressure is:

    a. Essential hypertension

    b. Rightsided heart failure

    c. Anxiety

    d. Valsalva maneuver

31. Typically, a grade 4 radial pulse could be described as:

    a. Absent

    b. Decreased or diminished

    c. Bounding

    d. Full or increased

32. True or false: It is okay for a patient to be supine when you palpate the arterial pulses.

    a. True

    b. False

33. The best spot to listen for mitral valve murmurs is:

    a. The cardiac apex

    b. Erb's point

    c. The tricuspid area

    d. Lateral wall

34. Which ov the following statements about the third heart sound is correct?

    a. It occurs at the beginning of ventricular systole.

    b. It may be a normal variant in young adults.

    c. It is best heard with the patient standing.

    d. It is best heard with the diaphragm of the stethoscope.

35. True or false: The fourth heart sound is a low-frequency sound and thus is best heard with the diaphragm of the stethoscope.

    a. True

    b. False

36. A murmur may be classified as low-, medium-, or high-pitched, depending on which of the following?

    a. The velocity of blood flow

    b. The age of the patient

    c. The point on the chest at which it is heard

    d. The area of origin

37. How is a click different from a murmur?

    a. Most clicks are sustained sounds.

    b. Clicks can be heard only in infants and children.

    c. Clicks are short, high-pitched sounds.

    d. Clicks occur as paired sounds.

38. True or false: Pericardial friction rubs are caused by abnormal movement of the diaphragm against the left ventricle.

    a. True

    b. False

CHAPTER 5

DIAGNOSTIC TESTING FOR CARDIAC DISEASES

CHAPTER OBJECTIVE

After studying this chapter, the reader will be able to discuss the information derived from the chest radiographs, ECG, stress tests, echocardiogram, imaging scans, cardiac catheterization, coronary angiogram, and electrophysiologic studies and to describe the nursing care of a patient undergoing these tests.

LEARNING OBJECTIVES

After studying this chapter, the reader should be able to

1. Describe two types of information about the heart that a plain chest radiograph can provide.

2. Specify nursing interventions for patients having ECG monitoring.

3. Name two criteria for ordering stress tests.

4. Name two absolute contraindications for stress testing.

5. State two reasons a stress test should be terminated.

6. Recognize a patient who would benefit from a dipyridamole thallium test rather than regular thallium testing.

7. Specify two reasons an echocardiogram may be ordered.

8. State two reasons nuclear imaging would be done.

9. Choose, from a list, an indication for magnetic resonance imaging.

10. Name three pressures obtained during cardiac catheterization.

11. Differentiate cardiac catheterization and coronary angiography.

12. Name one reason for electrophysiologic studies.

13. Choose appropriate nursing interventions for patients undergoing each of the aforementioned tests.

INTRODUCTION

A variety of diagnostic tests are available for accessing cardiovascular function. They range from simple screening tests, such as chest radiographs and ECG, available in most outpatient areas, to highly technical tests that use radionuclides and computerized analysis. The type of testing depends on the patient's clinical picture, the information sought, and the availability of equipment.

The ideal test is noninvasive, free of complications, inexpensive, and highly informative. Because no test has all these characteristics, diagnosing the presence or absence of disease requires that several tests be performed. When choosing a test and interpreting the results, the practitioner must be aware of the ability of the test to detect disease (sensitivity) and the ability of the test to exclude disease (specificity).

This chapter begins with the simpler tests and proceeds to more complex procedures. Each test is described in terms of how it is done and what it can tell about cardiovascular health. Tests are summarized in *Table 10* at the end of the chapter. Nursing care of the patient undergoing the test is discussed.

LABORATORY TESTS

Blood tests. No blood test can predict a patient's risk for CHD. However, several measurements, including plasma cholesterol levels and plasma glucose levels, can help the nurse develop a profile of a patient at risk. For most patients, a complete blood count is done. Most hospital and office practices measure serum glucose, blood urea nitrogen, uric acid, hemoglobin, cholesterol, liver enzymes, and creatinine, as well as plasma sodium and potassium levels. The following are tests that are particularly pertinent for the patient at risk of CHD.

Plasma cholesterol levels. Because the relationship between plasma cholesterol levels and risk for CHD is well-established in studies such as the Framingham study and the Pooling Project, measuring plasma cholesterol levels is an important step of any physical examination. As the AHA (1987) has pointed out, two levels of plasma cholesterol have emerged as guideposts to assist in managing patients. A cholesterol concentration in middle-aged adults below 200 mg/dL seems to be associated with a relatively low risk for CHD. However, the second level, a measurement over 240 mg/dL, approximately doubles the risk. Patients with values in the intermediate range, such as 200– 240 mg/dL, deserve counseling and attention but do not require intensive intervention and follow-up.

Plasma cholesterol and triglycerides should be measured at least every 5 years. In asymptomatic persons whose plasma total cholesterol level is below 200 mg/dL, no additional measurements are required for another 5 years. Even so, it is a good idea to point out the importance of a fat-modified diet, in which fat is limited to less than 30% of total calories. In addition, patients should attempt to keep saturated and polyunsaturated fats at a level of less than 10% (each) of total calories (AHA, 1987). Ideally, cholesterol levels should approximate 100 mg for every 1,000 calories and should not exceed 300 mg/ day.

For people whose adjusted levels of cholesterol are between 200 and 240 mg/dL on the first measurement, special attention should be turned to the possibility of other risk factors, such as smoking, hypertension, obesity, a family history of premature CHD and, clinical signs of CHD (Grundy et al., 1987).

When the initial plasma cholesterol level is greater than 240 mg/dL, plasma lipid and lipoprotein studies should be done. If a high concentration of cholesterol is confirmed and is not related to an elevated HDL level, the patient can be classified as having hypercholesterolemia. It is justifiable to have an age-adjusted definition of hypercholesterolemia to alert a young adult to a tendency to increased risk, but active intervention (medication) is rarely indicated for cholesterol levels below 240 mg/dL, regardless of age (Grundy et al., 1987). Appropriate laboratory tests will exclude secondary forms of hypercholesterolemia, such as hypothyroidism, nephrotic syndrome, or primary biliary cirrhosis. It is also a good idea to screen first-degree relatives for plasma lipid levels to detect genetic forms of hyperlipidemia, such as the relatively uncommon but severe metabolic disorder familial hypercholesterolemia, which is found in about 1 in 500 people.

When hypercholesterolemia is diagnosed, the first step should be to help patients modify their diet. If hypercholesterolemia does not respond within 2 or more months, physicians generally consider referral to a therapeutic dietitian for more intense dietary management and counseling. For some patients, drug therapy is required. However, this should not be attempted until dietary modification has been tried (AHA, 1987).

HDL cholesterol. Several environmental elements can cause reduced plasma levels of HDL cholesterol, including obesity, lack of exercise, and smoking (McGee & Gordon, 1976; Phillips, Havel, & Kane, 1981; Wolf & Grundy, 1983). Drugs commonly used to treat hypertension can also lower HDL levels, as will androgens, progestational agents, and anabolic steroids. Hypertriglyceridemia and hypercholesterolemia often produce low levels of plasma HDL.

Several approaches have been helpful for increasing HDL levels, including weight reduction; correcting hypertriglyceridemia or hypercholesterolemia; frequent, vigorous exercise; stopping smoking; keeping alcohol use at moderate levels; and use of estrogens. Another method is to try to double efforts to lower total cholesterol and LDL cholesterol or to reduce plasma levels of triglycerides.

Plasma glucose levels. The link between fasting hyperglycemia (diabetes mellitus) and risk of CHD is well established. Thus, measurement of blood glucose levels should be part of any laboratory workup. Fasting blood glucose levels should be obtained at 5-year intervals in people between the ages of 20 and 60, at 2.5-year intervals in those between 61 and 75, and optionally after age 75. These recommendations generally apply to people who are nonobese, or those who weigh less than 110% of desirable body weight (Grundy et al., 1987). For those who are mild to moderately obese, or 110–130% above ideal body weight, testing should be done every 2.5 years after age 45. Markedly obese patients should be tested annually after they are 50 years old.

Diabetes mellitus can be diagnosed when a patient has elevated plasma glucose levels after an overnight fast. That is, after they have two values of fasting blood glucose greater than 140 mg/dL. Any obese, middle-aged person is a candidate for diabetes, because 80% of those who acquire diabetes are obese. Obesity enhances peripheral resistance to the action of insulin, which probably contributes greatly to the development of diabetes.

CHEST RADIOGRAPH

Radiologic studies can provide detailed information about the heart's structure and function that cannot be supplied by any other diagnostic method. The routine chest radiograph, included in nearly every complete physical examination, can indicate the presence of heart disease and sometimes can show a specific heart problem. Furthermore, it can be used to determine the size and shape of the heart. Because nearly every person has had a chest radiograph obtained, such radiographs form an important baseline measurement. They may also provide the first evidence of unsuspected heart disease. The chest radiograph is still the most cost-effective, available, simple, and reliable initial screening tool in the evaluation of cardiovascular disease.

In a normal adult, a chest radiograph shows a heart diameter equal to 50% or less of the diameter of the chest. Short or obese adults may have a higher ratio. The difference between a normal heart and a greatly enlarged one is usually obvious. Minor increases in size are more difficult to see.

Normal findings. A complete radiologic study of the heart involves four views of the chest: frontal, lateral, 60° right anterior oblique, and 45° left anterior oblique views. For many practical reasons, the heart cannot be studied from one aspect or view. On a chest radiograph, the heart appears to be relatively homogeneous because many of its structures (such as the myocardium and the valves) have the same radiodensity as blood, and the cardiac shadows blend into one another. In fact, intracardiac lesions cannot be visualized unless they are calcified.

The opposite is true of the contours of the heart, which are well outlined because they contrast with the lungs, which are radiolucent because of the air they contain. The only areas of the heart that can be seen well are chambers and vessels that form a border on any particular view. In addition, because the heart is a three-dimensional structure, it must be viewed from several different aspects to bring each of the heart chambers and the vessels into clear view or profile. In addition, for the examiner to see the posterior border of the heart, the patient must swallow radiopaque material so that the esophagus can be differentiated from the heart.

All chest radiographs are taken with the radiographic tube about 6 ft (1.8 m) away from the heart. The posteroanterior view is taken with the patient standing close to the film with the arms extended over the head and centered over the body. The patient is told to take a deep breath and hold it while the radiograph is obtained. For lateral radiographs, the patient again holds the arms over the head and inspires deeply. Each view shows specific views of the heart, lungs, and great vessels. The sum of all views gives the best picture of the patient's heart and lungs.

When a patient is too ill to be transported to the radiology department, a portable chest radiograph can be obtained at the bedside. Although it is similar to the posteroanterior view, the anteroposterior view is not as clear as that obtained with the patient standing with arms extended over the head. For the best possible radiograph, the patient should be upright in bed (to allow the diaphragm to drop, promoting optimal lung expansion), and mechanical devices should be moved out of the line of the radiograph as much as possible.

Abnormal findings. The posteroanterior view shows enlargement of the heart chamber and pulmonary congestion. For further clarification of cardiac enlargement, an ECG is obtained to determine the presence of chamber hypertrophy. The lateral view is used to assess the size of the left ventricle and the left atrium. The right anterior oblique view is used to assess enlargement of the right ventricular outflow tract and the main pulmonary artery. The left anterior oblique view can show left-sided lesions, coarctation of the aorta, patent ductus arteriosus, and dilatation of the ascending aorta (Sokolow, McIlroy, & Cheitlin, 1990).

Frequently, patients with ischemic disease have normal findings on chest radiographs. Even so, chest radiographs can be helpful in such patients because the radiographs can show congestive changes in the lungs and can be used to estimate the degree of pulmonary venous hypertension. Chest radiographs also provide a baseline that can be compared with subsequent radiographs to show a change in left ventricular contour or size and, occasionally, to reveal the complications of myocardial disease (calcifications, aneurysm, post-MI syndrome, mitral insufficiency, and septal perforation, among others).

Left atrial enlargement most often is due to mitral valve disease. The left atrium enlarges disproportionately and fills in the "waist" of the heart. Right atrial enlargement may be due to an atrial septal defect. Other possibilities include tricuspid insufficiency or stenosis.

Evaluation of the pulmonary vasculature also provides information about the circulation and left ventricular function. The size of the central pulmonary arteries (the left pulmonary artery and its hilar branches) gives an index of the pulmonary artery pressure. Normally, the larger peripheral vessels are in the lower part of the lung. The sizes of the more peripheral pulmonary vessels are reflections of pulmonary blood volume and also give a rough estimate of the pulmonary blood pressure and flow. When the main pulmonary arteries are dilated, and normal variations because of aging and other factors are ruled out, right ventricular hypertrophy and/or dilatation is almost always present.

ELECTROCARDIOGRAM

For detailed instruction on the normal ECG and recognition of dysrhythmias, see *Coronary Care Modules* by Marlene Pechan, published by Williams & Wilkins, or any other basic book on electrocardiography. This section is intended to describe the ECG as a diagnostic tool for cardiovascular disease.

The ECG is one of the most useful clinical tools used to uncover anatomic, metabolic, ionic, and hemodynamic changes in the heart. It often is an independent marker of myocardial disease. Sometimes it is the only way to detect asymptomatic heart disease. The ECG is the gold standard for diagnosing arrhythmias, because no other method can detect them with the same level of sensitivity and specificity. With the data obtained from ECGs, you can detect ischemia, injury, infarcts, cardiac arrhythmias, cardiac enlargement, electrolyte disturbances, pericarditis, and the effects of some drugs.

Intermittent 12-lead ECGs are done in routine health examinations, as part of preoperative assessments, when a patient experiences chest pain, and on similar occasions. These ECGs may show a dysrhythmia or an episode of myocardial ischemia. They also can be used to track the progress of an MI. However, the abnormality being sought may not show up on this type of ECG. To increase the likelihood of discovering an abnormality, coronary care units have been established where the patient is monitored continuously on a cardiac monitor.

Continuous ECG monitoring usually shows only 1 or 2 of the standard 12 leads available in an ECG. The practitioner can select which leads to monitor on the basis of the patient's history and the problem being examined. When an incident suggests a coronary problem (chest pain or dysrhythmias), a 12-lead ECG can be done, to show cardiac electrical activity from a variety of views. ECGs can be done repeatedly as the precipitating incident resolves spontaneously or in response to medical treatment.

For both the 12-lead ECG and continuous ECG monitoring, the testing procedure should be explained to patients, and they should be assured that they will feel no discomfort. They will need to remain still for a few seconds during the actual recording of the rhythm strip during the 12-lead ECG. They will be able to move about in bed or in their room within the limits of the monitoring device when continuous ECG monitoring is used. Patients should know that monitor alarms will ring periodically but generally do not mean that a serious problem exists. Usually the alarm rings because of a loose monitor electrode, a lead falling off, or mechanical or electrical interference with the signal. These situations can be remedied quickly and painlessly by the nurse.

Another method of continuous ECG monitoring is the use of a Holter monitor. This is a portable monitor that patients can wear as they go about their daily activities. Patients are given a log in which to record the exact time of day (as seen on a clock on the battery pack), the activity they are doing, and how they are feeling. This monitoring goes on for 12- to 24-hr, and then the equipment is removed. A technician reviews the 12 to 24 hr tape of the patient's ECG for abnormalities and submits abnormal findings to a cardiologist for analysis. Abnormal findings can be correlated with patients' daily activities and with symptoms. The value of the Holter monitor recording depends largely on how well patients record their activities and symptoms. Therefore, good education of the patient about this procedure is vital.

EXERCISE TESTING

Stress exercise tests provide a key diagnostic tool for determining diagnostically and prognostically important cardiovascular abnormalities while a patient is tested in the controlled and safe setting of a cardiovascular testing laboratory. The cornerstone of modern stress testing is based on the discovery that exercise in patients with coronary heart disease produces ST-segment depression on ECGs (Ellestad, 1986).

By using controlled exercise tests, usually involving walking on a treadmill, you can detect mechanical abnormalities, such as a low peak heart rate, low blood pressure, reduced workload, ischemic abnormalities such as angina pectoris, and electrical abnormalities such as premature ventricular contractions (PVCs). In many institutions, exercise stress testing is teamed with myocardial imaging, so that an image of the heart can be obtained along with stress ECGs. These tests may also be useful in the diagnosis of labile hypertension.

Stress tests also are useful for estimating cardiac prognosis. Studies of cardiac function during exercise have shown that the prognosis is good for patients whose mechanical response to exercise (peak treadmill workload, heart rate, and cardiac output) is well preserved despite moderate-to-severe anatomic coronary disease.

Indications for exercise testing. Exercise testing is used mainly to diagnose overt or latent CHD, especially angina pectoris, and to differentiate the causes of inexplicable chest pain.

Another important purpose of exercise testing is to test the functional capacity of cardiac patients, such as those who have had an MI or have undergone coronary artery bypass surgery. For example, patients who have recently recovered from an MI are often candidates for low-level exercise testing. Monitoring the heart during exercise allows the examiner to determine how well the heart is functioning and also helps in the design of a management program for the patient.

A person's functional capacity easily can be evaluated by determining the maximal amount of exercise he or she can tolerate, which can be expressed as multiples of the resting metabolic activity, or METs. The term MET (metabolic equivalent unit) is used to describe the energy required to perform a specific action, based on the amount of oxygen consumed at 3.5 ml/kg/min. For example, 1 MET is the energy cost, or the amount of oxygen used per minute by a person who is sitting quietly. The MET is a useful way to measure a patient's peak workload.

Exercise stress testing also provides a way to test healthy asymptomatic persons for any sport or occupation that may demand unusual levels of physical activity. Often, the results of stress ECGs can be good motivating tools to help encourage sedentary persons to slowly but surely build their strength and to adopt a healthier and more active lifestyle. These tests also are used for research and as a screening tool for life insurance companies.

Exercise testing modes. Many exercise testing modes are available, including treadmill tests, step tests, cycle ergometry, and dynamic upper extremity testing. Treadmill testing is the most popular and widely used method for exercise testing in the United States, whereas cycle ergometry is more popular in other countries. Technical improvements such as quieter treadmills, low-impedance ECG electrodes, and signal averaging of the QRS complex have minimized earlier disadvantages of treadmill testing, such as motion artifacts or difficulties recording blood pressure with a sphygmomanometer. Treadmill testing also has been more effective then cycle ergometry because Americans are less familiar with cycling than with walking and climbing, and their exercise tolerance often is limited because of weakness of the quadriceps or because of knee problems.

Cycle ergometry may be the test of choice for obese or poorly coordinated persons who cannot perform even low-intensity treadmill exercises. In addition, cycle ergometry is the only method of exercise used with radionuclide ventriculography and the only practical way to use dynamic exercise during cardiac catheterization.

Both cycle ergometry and treadmill testing are comparable in sensitivity and specificity. Peak heart rates and peak systolic and diastolic pressure are lower with treadmill testing.

Exercise Test Protocols

Selecting the proper protocol for exercise ECG testing is extremely important because the sensitivity of the test is directly influenced by the type of protocol used (Chung, 1986). A variety of exercise tests besides the treadmill test are available, including the Master's Two-Step, the Harvard Step Test, and others. This text concentrates on treadmill testing because it is by far the most popular test and the most widely used in the United States. Treadmill testing has a number of advantages over step testing, including the ability to adjust the speed and grade of the treadmill to match the ability of the subject.

In some centers, exercise testing is continued until the patient has significant symptoms, such as chest pain. Others halt treadmill testing when the submaximal heart rate, or 85–90% of the predicted maximal heart rate, is reached, whether or not the patient reports any symptoms or whether or not any ECG abnormalities are seen.

Symptom-limited testing usually is preferred to heart-rate-limited or "submaximal" testing because the greater heart rate, higher blood pressure, and greater workload that can be elicited by symptom-limited testing are more likely to uncover diagnostically and prognostically important cardiac abnormalities. Symptom-limited testing is continued to the point of limiting symptoms of angina pectoris, generalized fatigue, dyspnea, and local

muscle fatigue or until other abnormalities appear that may make it unsafe to continue exercise. These abnormalities might include marked ischemic ST segment depression of 0.3 mV or more; exercise-induced hypotension (a fall of 10 mm Hg or more in systolic pressure compared with the blood pressure measured in an earlier stage of exercise); or complex ventricular ectopic beats, such as three or more consecutive PVCs.

Exercise testing can be continued as long as the patient does not complain of chest pain, shortness of breath, marked fatigue, or feelings of near-syncope. When exercise stress testing is terminated on the basis of the predicted heart rate alone, the cardiac workload is often insufficient; in many physically inactive persons, a disproportionately rapid heart rate develops with minimal amounts of exercise because of their poor physical conditioning. False-negative results are common under such circumstances (Chung, 1986).

Ideally, the exercise ECG protocol should be closely matched to each patient's anticipated physical capacity. It should include an activity that can be performed by sedentary, poorly developed, and underconditioned persons as well as by trained athletes. Workloads should be increased gradually, not abruptly, and continued long enough to produce a near-physiologic steady state. The protocol should not cause physical or mental stress beyond tolerable workloads. Patients should be monitored continually with at least a two-channel recorder and 1-min interval recordings of rhythm strips throughout the entire exercise periods and for at least 6–8 min after the exercise program. In addition, the subject's blood pressure should be measured periodically (at 1- to 3-min intervals) before, during, and after exercise. The stress test should be halted when abnormal signs, symptoms, and ECG readings occur.

Several of the most commonly used exercise test formats are the Harvard Step Test and the

Bruce, Balke, and Naughton protocols. Because all protocols elicit similar peak oxygen consumption levels, the selection of a particular protocol usually is guided by the examiner's evaluation of the estimated effort tolerance of each patient. The Naughton test, for example, requires a low initial workload and small increments in workload thereafter and often is used for testing patients who recently have had an MI, have had bypass surgery, or have angina or other symptoms that make higher workloads intolerable. The Bruce protocol, in contrast, is best for patients who have no known limitations.

The goal of all protocols is to produce a symptom-limited response within 6–15 min after exercise begins. A briefer test may miss ischemic responses. A longer one may be limited by muscular fatigue rather then myocardial ischemia.

Early low-level testing protocols for post-MI patients. Low-level protocols are often designed for patients who have recovered from acute MIs. It is now common to order modified stress tests for MI patients before the patients are discharged from the hospital after an acute MI (Ellestad, 1986). Others are offered testing 4–6 weeks after recovery. These low-level stress tests help detect patients at high risk by eliciting ECG abnormalities, cardiac symptoms, or arrhythmias provoked at minimal workloads.

Contraindications to stress testing. Relative and absolute contraindications to stress testing exist. Absolute contraindications can include noncardiac reasons, such as serious pulmonary or renal disease. Overall, exercise testing has been associated with a low prevalence of morbidity or mortality when patients are selected carefully and when the test is supervised directly by an experienced cardiologist. Here is a short list of conditions that are currently considered absolute contraindications:

1. Acute MI

2. Unstable or crescendo angina

3. Serious cardiac arrhythmias, such as ventricular tachycardia, rapid atrial arrhythmias, or second- or third-degree heart blocks

4. Acute myocarditis or pericarditis, subacute bacterial endocarditis, acute rheumatic fever

5. Left main coronary disease

6. Any acute or serious noncardiac problem

7. Severe physical handicaps, such as severe arthritis, spinal deformity, or amputation

8. Serious or acute pulmonary, renal, hepatic, or malignant illness

9. Severe anemia

10. High fever

11. Mental instability or lack of cooperation

The following are relative contraindications to stress testing:

1. Suspected left main coronary disease

2. Congestive heart failure

3. Clinically significant noncardiac disorders

4. Idiopathic hypertrophic subaortic stenosis

5. Significant physical handicaps

6. Debilitated or elderly patients

7. Moderate-to-severe hypertension

8. Pulmonary hypertension

9. Moderate aortic stenosis

10. Clinically significant tachycardias (frequent multifocal PVCs)

11. Marked bradyarrhythmias

12. Drug-induced electrolyte imbalance

13. Use of various noncardiac agents, such as alcohol, tranquilizers, or analgesics

14. Fixed-rate pacemaker

Symptomatic end points. Symptom-limited exercise testing is preferable to submaximal testing under almost every circumstance, except very soon after an MI. To make sure patients are safe while they are walking on the treadmill, watch for signs such as puffing, dizziness, lack of coordination, pallor, or cold sweat. Patients should also be told before the test that they can stop at any point, although they are encouraged to try to reach or exceed the maximal predicted heart rate (Ellestad, 1986).

Stress testing should be stopped immediately when any of the following occurs:

- The patient asks that the test be stopped.

- Blood pressure or heart rate falls during increasing workloads.

- The patient complains of severe chest pain, ataxia, vertigo, gait disturbances, fatigue, or feeling faint.

- The patient is confused or has pallor or cyanosis or looks "clammy."

- The examiner notices several (three or more) serious arrhythmias grouped together: PVCs, ventricular tachycardia, or ventricular fibrillation.

- Atrial flutter is detected.

- The patient has musculoskeletal pain (arthritis or claudication).

- Extreme elevations in systolic and diastolic pressure are recorded, and the patient has a headache or blurred vision.

- The patient reports progressive anginal pain (e.g., grade 3 pain when the worst pain the patient has before experienced has been grade 4).

For some persons, any test or medical procedure will induce a high level of emotional stress. The nurse can differentiate this type of stress from exercise-induced changes by observing several factors. These types of patients often have high pulse rates during the early warm-up stages. However, once they become acclimated and begin to use physical effort, the pulse rate tends to level off rather than continue upward, because the effect of exertion offsets the effect of the early stress

(Levitas, 1979). It is important to monitor patients during the warm-up period just as closely as during the later phases of the test because the patient's coronary status may be so poor that he or she will have changes even during the warm-up period. The key to safety is to watch carefully and communicate with the patient during each phase of the test.

Part of monitoring involves watching for angina pectoris, dyspnea and fatigue, leg fatigue, claudication, and joint pain and measuring the blood pressure at regular intervals. Blood pressure should be measured at the end of each 3-min stage of exercise and at 1-min intervals when the blood pressure does not rise by 10 mm Hg compared with an earlier stage of exercise. A fall of 10 mm Hg in systolic pressure compared with a recording made during an earlier stage of exercise or rest is an indication that the test should be stopped. Falling pressure during exercise may be an indication of severe ischemic left ventricular dysfunction, especially if the patient also has angina pectoris or if it occurs at a low workload. In contrast, an exercise-induced fall in blood pressure in a patient receiving a ß-blocker or hypotension that occurs only at a high workload and heart rate, especially without any signs of angina pectoris, may have little significance.

Excessive blood pressure, or pressure higher than 280 mm Hg, is rarely reason enough to stop exercise. The elevated pressure has not been linked to any cardiac complications from exercise testing.

Complications. Serious complications resulting from exercise testing are relatively infrequent. Scherer and Kaltenbach (1979) reported on 750,000 patients with CHD who had undergone stress tests. The reported mortality rate was only 2 in 100,000. Various cardiac arrhythmias are the most common complications of exercise stress testing. Ventricular tachycardia, fibrillation, and flutter during and after exercise are the most serious cardiac rhythm problems, because they may lead to sudden death. Such ventricular tachyarrhythmias are often started by multifocal PVCs, the R-on-T phenomenon, and grouped PVCs (Chung, 1986). Bradyarrhythmias are uncommon and usually signal a serious outcome. Sick sinus syndrome should be suspected when the heart rate response to exercise is inadequate without any drug effect.

Angina pectoris and MI are two other possible complications of exercise testing. One of the most crucial points in diagnosing angina pectoris involves linking chest discomfort to ST segment depression during or after exercise. The chances of inducing angina by exercise ECG testing are greater when (a) the patient is known to have CHD affecting a number of vessels, (b) the test is given to patients soon after an acute MI, or (c) the exercise protocol calls for excessive workloads.

Congestive heart failure is another complication that may occur during stress testing. When myocardial ischemia is present, left ventricular compliance is reduced. Consider the possibility of congestive heart failure when paroxysmal cough develops during or soon after the exercise session in any patient with known or suspected CHD. This cough may be due to acute pulmonary congestion.

Hypotension or hypertension also may occur during or after exercise. Systolic blood pressure that increases more than 220 mm Hg during exercise is an abnormal finding. Hypotension or no change in blood pressure during testing is a far more serious problem than hypertension. Exercise-induced hypotension is most often noted in persons with advanced CHD affecting several vessels, and it frequently accompanies serious ventricular arrhythmias and marked ST segment depression (depression 2 mm or more horizontal to downsloping).

Elderly patients may lose their balance during the test, leading to musculoskeletal trauma. To counteract the possibility of falling, all patients should wear sturdy rubber-soled shoes, and the test should never be given while the patient is barefoot. Also, atherosclerosis is a systemic disease and may cause numerous systemic signs and symptoms as well as acting as a stressor on cardiac muscle. Peripheral claudication may be a problem and may lead to early termination of the stress test. Peripheral claudication usually improves once the patient rests.

Proper selection of patients is crucial. As always, the benefits of exercise stress testing must be weighed against the potential risks, especially in high-risk subjects. The second most important factor in the patient's safety, after proper selection of patients, is early detection of incipient left ventricular failure (indicated by a falling systolic pressure or cerebrovascular insufficiency shown by a staggering gait or mental confusion).

The safety of exercise testing can be improved by making adequate provisions for prompt cardiac resuscitation in the event of exercise-induced cardiac arrest. Specially trained nurses or physician's assistants can supervise stress testing in low-risk patients, but those who may be at high risk, such as those who are being tested 10–14 days or sooner after an MI, must be tested while a physician is present, in case they encounter difficulties.

Several pieces of equipment also should be available in case a patient has problems during a stress test. The following should be immediately at hand: a direct-current defibrillator (frequently tested), oral and tracheal airways, an oxygen supply, a hand respirator, a cut-down tray, and a laryngoscope. Full emergency resuscitation facilities usually are provided in the testing laboratory. All staff members must be well trained in cardiopulmonary resuscitation and advanced cardiac life support.

Many researchers have shown that exercise stress testing is a safe procedure when patients are selected carefully. Stress testing is not for everyone, and some patients should never have exercise testing.

Test Results

Normal physiologic changes. Several normal physiologic changes occur during an exercise stress test. Blood pressure and heart rate gradually rise, and the QT interval is shortened. Functional ST segment depression of 2 mm occurs, with a duration shorter than 0.06 sec. Other normal changes include labile T wave change; a slight reduction of the height of the R wave; downward displacement of the PR segment because of prominent T wave height; peaking and tall P waves during very rapid heart rate; and minor signs and symptoms such as dyspnea, fatigue, and sweating. *Figure 9* shows a typical ECG wave form.

The heart rate response is the best indicator of the extent of exertion. One of the most widely accepted ways to estimate the maximum rate that can be obtained for an individual patient is to deduct the patient's age from 220–230 (beats per minute). Well-conditioned persons may have lower heart rates. In fact, generally lowered heart rates are used as a measurement of improved physical conditioning after physical fitness programs (Ellestad, 1986).

Although there has been much interest in measuring oxygen consumption in patients undergoing stress tests, this is an expensive, time-consuming procedure that probably should not be included in a routine stress test. In addition, patients often are bothered by the mouthpiece and noseclip required during testing (Ellestad, 1986).

Abnormal responses. Abnormal responses include changes in the ECG such as ST segment alterations, cardiac arrhythmias, inversion of T waves, increased R wave height, slowing of the heart rate, marked hypertension, severe chest pain, dyspnea, pallor, cyanosis, third or fourth heart sounds, murmurs, precordial bulging, and pulsus aternans.

Exercise testing usually uncovers three major types of cardiac abnormalities: myocardial ischemia, left ventricular dysfunction, and ventricular ectopic activity. These three findings often are interrelated. For example ST segment displacement and/or angina often is accompanied by poor exercise tolerance, which reflects exercise-induced left ventricular dysfunction *(Figure 10)*.

The criteria most often used to diagnose exercise-induced myocardial ischemia are a flat or downsloping ST segment of 1 mm or more (Chung, 1986), an up sloping ST segment depression 2 mm or more beyond 0.08 sec from the J-point during or after exercise, and a horizontal or upsloping ST segment elevation of 1 mm or more during or after exercise. The significance of these findings is modified by such factors as the heart rate and workload at which the downsloping segment occurred, whether the patient also has exercise-induced angina or hypotension, the peak heart rate and workload that was achieved, and the persistence of signs and symptoms during recovery. Traditionally, the horizontal (square-wave) ST segment depression during or after exercise has been the most reliable ECG finding for a normal ECG stress test.

A number of factors can cause falsely normal or falsely abnormal findings. Among these are use of digitalis, antidepressants, or ß-blockers; inadequate exercise; and improper placement of leads. Certain groups of patients are more likely to have false-positive results: young women, people 20–25 years old, and pilots. Borderline tests are more common in middle-aged women than in middle-aged men. The causes for these phenomena are still being explored.

Exercise-induced ST segment elevation usually occurs in one of two settings: in ECG leads showing Q waves at rest (reflecting abnormalities in wall motion and or/peripheral ischemia), and in ECG leads reflecting severe transmural exercise-

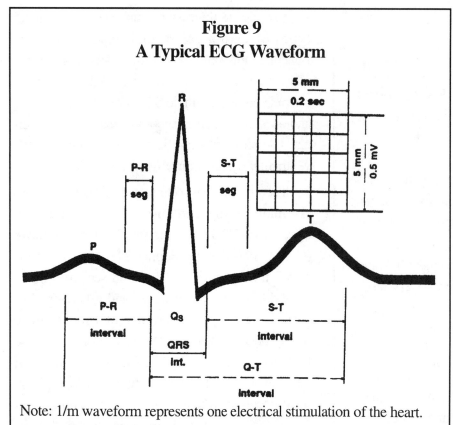

Figure 9
A Typical ECG Waveform

Note: 1/m waveform represents one electrical stimulation of the heart.

Preparing the Patient for the Test

It is essential to obtain informed consent with a form signed by the patient and witnessed by the physician before the patient is tested. The form advises the patient about the test and the slight risks of being tested. Before the test, the patient should be given a thorough explanation of how the stress test is performed and how the test results are interpreted. The history helps exclude those who are at high risk.

Preparations for the test. Patients should not smoke cigarettes or eat for at least 2 hr before the test. They should wear comfortable clothing and rubber-soled shoes for good traction. Slippers may be comfortable, but they are unacceptable for the test. Men can wear gym shorts, bermuda shorts, or lightweight, loose trousers. Women should wear a bra; a short-sleeved, loose-fitting blouse that buttons in the front; and slacks, shorts, or pajama bottoms.

Subjects should plan to be in the exercise laboratory for 60–90 min. The laboratory should be kept at a comfortable temperature, (between 68°F and 74°F) with moderate humidity (between 40% and 60%). If the stress test is being done to evaluate functional effects of ischemic heart disease, patients should continue to take most of their medications. If the stress test is being done for diagnostic reasons, such as to evaluate the cause of chest pain, all cardiac medications may be withdrawn before testing so that the ST segment response to exercise is not affected. Generally, patients are advised that medications such as digitalis, propra-

induced myocardial ischemia associated with critically severe, fixed coronary stenosis or coronary artery spasm. Such abnormalities are generally detected in leads V_1 and aVL. Isolated T wave alterations, as in direction or shape during or after exercise, are considered to be of no significance and to have no diagnostic implications (Chung, 1986). Thus, most exercise laboratories ignore isolated T wave alterations.

The peak workload attained during symptom-limited exercise testing is a clinically important measure of functional limitation due to cardiac or noncardiac conditions, such as obesity, orthopedic or pulmonary vascular disease, general debilitation, and deconditioning. When the noncardiac causes are ruled out, a low peak exercise workload during symptom-limited testing usually represents either fixed left ventricular dysfunction from infarction or other myocardial disease, exercise-induced myocardial ischemia, or the functional consequences of valvular or pericardial disease.

nolol, and diuretics may interfere with the test, and they should check with their primary care physician about continuing or discontinuing such drugs before the test. Because they may not be familiar with the trade names or generic names of their medications, these can be described as "heart pills" or "water pills."

Patients also should be warned that they will be short of breath and fatigued during the test, particularly when they reach higher levels of effort. Reassurance and encouragement during the test help. Many testing centers have the patient rest comfortably supine for at least 5–10 min before the exercise session begins. Immediately after the test, patients should be reexamined with cardiac auscultation in the left lateral decubitus position to detect any exercise-induced ischemic abnormalities such as new S_3 of S_4 gallops, mitral regurgitation murmurs (which may reflect papillary muscle dysfunction), or left ventricular aneurysmal bulging.

Stress Testing with Radionuclides

Thallium studies. Stress testing with radionuclides is done to assess myocardial perfusion and ventricular function. It does not detect and measure specific obstructions in the coronary arteries. It is helpful in assessing patients who have had an MI, screening for high-risk patients (those with left-sided main disease and three-vessel disease), and evaluating progress from cardiac rehabilitation programs. For patients with inconclusive or normal results for treadmill stress tests, nuclear imaging can predict sites of coronary artery disease. Because it is more sensitive and specific then treadmill exercise testing, it can add more information to positive results on a stress test (D. Miller et al., 1988).

The radionuclide used is thallium-201. It is extracted from the blood by the myocardium in the same way that potassium is extracted. As the radionuclide first passes through the myocardium, 85% is taken up by the cells. Poor uptake (indicat-

ing poor myocardial perfusion) shows up as a cold spot on the scan.

Exercise usually is performed on a standard treadmill or bicycle ergometer, according to standard exercise protocols, such as the Bruce protocol. At peak exercise, when the pulse rate is at its highest, and when the subject states that he or she is nearing the limits of exercise tolerance, 3 ml of saline containing 2–3 mCi of thallium-201 is injected into a free-flowing intravenous line in a large vein in the forearm or upper arm of the subject. The subject is advised to continue to exercise for 60 sec after the injection, to make certain that maximum coronary blood flow is maintained while the thallium is flowing through the myocardium.

As soon as the ECG has returned to baseline after exercise, the patient is positioned under the gamma camera. Ideally, the time between injection and scan should be less than 5 min. A longer delay allows the thallium to redistribute undetected, and the sensitivity of the test is diminished (D. Miller et al., 1988). Thallium tends to leave the heart muscle quickly, and the scan must be obtained at an optimal time.

Scans are obtained with the patient at rest and after injection of the radionuclide at peak exercise because perfusion of the left ventricle at rest in a patient without previous infarction is usually normal even when severe coronary narrowing is present. The radionuclide redistributes within an hour, and imaging should be completed within 45 min after injection, if possible (Warren & Lewis, 1985). Generally, two 45° views are obtained: an anterior view or a 45° left anterior oblique view and either a left lateral view or steep (70°) left anterior oblique view. With the anterior view, the examiner can assess the activity of thallium in the lung. The 45° view allows assessment of all three coronary areas simultaneously. The 70° left anterior oblique or left lateral view enables the examiner to see the inferior and posterior walls of the heart.

Figure 10
Abnormal Responses to Stress Exercise Testing

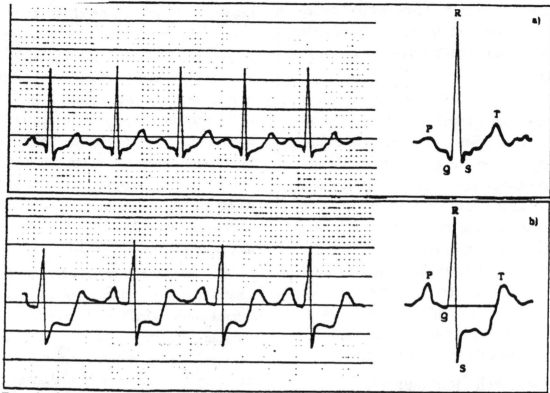

Example of a) normal and b) ischemic response to exercise. For the purpose of determining the ECG response to exercise, the PQ segment must be taken as the isoelectric line.

Magnitude of ST depression	Electrocardiographic appearance	Sensitivity	Specificity
0.5 mm		84%	57%
1.0 mm		62%	89%
1.5 mm		48%	100%

The sensitivity and specificity of different magnitudes of ST segment depression. The actual percentage will vary from group to group, but the relative differences should remain roughly the same.

From: Martin CM, McConahay DR Circulation 1972: 46: 956-62. By permission of the American Heart Association Inc..

Preparation of the patient. Patients generally are advised that they should have a light breakfast and avoid strenuous exercise before they take the test. If the patient is receiving antianginal medications such as ß-blockers or calcium blockers, these may be withheld before the test by the physician's instruction. Diabetic patients can eat if necessary.

During the stress test, the patient's ECG, blood pressure, and clinical signs and symptoms must be monitored, just as with the standard exercise stress test (Ellestad, 1986). The test is ended (a) when the patient attains sex- and age-predicted target heart rates, (b) the patient has to stop the exercise because of symptoms, (c) the ST segment changes more than 3 mm, (d) systolic pressure drops by more than 20 mm Hg, or (5) significant ventricular tachycardia or fibrillation develops.

Three to four hours after exercise, patients undergo redistribution imaging. Between the two imaging sessions, they should avoid excessive exertion or foods high in sugar, because both of these may increase myocardial clearance of thallium. The remarkable views of the heart obtained with nuclear scans show areas of the heart that are not receiving adequate perfusion.

Dipyridamole thallium studies. Some patients, such as those who have orthopedic problems or who recently had a stroke, are not candidates for exercise testing. However, a form of thallium scanning is available for them.

Dipyridamole (Persantine) thallium studies are a good alternative for these patients. Dipyridamole acts as a potent vasodilator, often increasing coronary blood flow more than it can be increased with maximal exercise regiments (Chapmen et al., 1979) Coronary blood flow is increased twofold to threefold in areas supplied by normal coronary arteries. Areas with diseased coronary arteries are unable to increase their flow, thus increasing the discrepancy between normal and abnormal coronary artery flow (Sokolow et al., 1990).

Dipyridamole thallium studies are safe although a number of transient side effects such as headache (20% of patients), chest pain (18%), dizziness, and gastrointestinal disturbances are reported. In addition, up to a third of patients experience the "coronary steal" phenomenon, in which the flow to ischemic regions is reduced, causing ST segment changes and angina (Leppo et al., 1982).

Preparation of the patient. Before the test, patients are advised to avoid coffee, tea, aminophylline, and other xanthine-containing substances, which would antagonize the effects of dipyridamole. They fast for 2 hr, then a free-running intravenous line is established, and 0.5–1.0 mg/kg of dipyridamole is infused over 5 min. Baseline ECGs, blood pressure, and heart rate are recorded,

and these are monitored at 1-min intervals during the study. After the agent is infused, patients can sit up, if they wish, and do a hand-grip exercise. Approximately 10 min after infusion, the patient lies down, and 2 mCi of thallium is infused intravenously. The first scan is made within 15 min after the initial infusion of dipyridamole.

If the patient has significant angina with prolonged ECG evidence of myocardial ischemia, 100 mg of aminophylline is infused slowly intravenously. This reverses the relative flow changes induced by dipyridamole, so at least one image set should be obtained before the aminophylline is given.

Results of thallium scans. The scans obtained during exercise stress testing or with dipyridamole thallium studies are interpreted by three or more observers at a computer console. Usually, to avoid bias, the observers do not compare results with clinical information. They examine the initial images and the delayed images, looking for signs of redistribution or partial or complete disappearance of the initial defect (D. Miller et al., 1988). They then examine the myocardial segments and overall myocardial size. Dilatation during exercise is a sign of myocardial dysfunction or failure. When no change in size between the first and the delayed image sets is seen, the patient usually has a fixed defect, such as a myocardial scar.

ECHOCARDIOGRAPHY

Ultrasound is one of the oldest and newest imaging techniques. It could be thought of as the oldest because a primitive form of ultrasound, echolocation, is used by many animal species, such as bats, dolphins, and whales. It is also one of the newest imaging techniques available for studying the heart, because it really has been refined only during the past two decades. During the past 15 years or so, the development of diagnostic ultrasound techniques has revolutionized the diagnosis of heart disease. It is a powerful, noninvasive technique that allows the examiner to obtain information about the heart's structure and function, including the cardiac chambers, walls, and valves, areas that may be difficult to study with ordinary chest radiographs.

The basis for ultrasound came from the development of radar and sonar during World War II. Ultrasound uses pulse-echo techniques to define accurately anatomic images of tissue and fluid interfaces within the body. That is, it sends out a signal that strikes, then bounces back from various tissues of the body. The information then is recorded on videotape and on paper. Ultrasound also can be used to show motion, is simple to perform, and eliminates some of the unfavorable aspects of other examinations, such as exposure to radioneuclides and contrast materials.

Echocardiography can be defined as the use of ultrasound to examine the heart. The upper limit of audible sound is 20,000 cycles/sec, or 20 kHz. The sonic frequency used for echocardiography ranges from 1 million to 7 million cycles/sec, or 1–7 MHz. These ranges are even higher in children.

Unlike x-ray studies, which use radiation to study internal structures, ultrasound creates an image by reflecting sound waves off an object. These sound waves penetrate soft tissues and are reflected at interfaces between blood and heart muscle or valves. They do not penetrate bone or air-containing lung tissue. High-frequency sound waves (10 MHz) penetrate poorly and are good for visualizing surface structures. Low-frequency sound waves (2 MHz) penetrate well to 20 cm and are good for deeper structures. The sound waves go through the transducer located on the outside of the chest and are processed electronically to form images on a screen. For detailed studies of the atrium well, the patient swallows a small transducer and the data are gathered via a transducer placed in the esophagus, which is close to the atrium.

Indications for ultrasound. Echocardiography is a relatively inexpensive way to evaluate left ventricular function in patients with known and significant cardiovascular disease.

Patients who are fairly ill and who are showing signs and symptoms of low cardiac output or congestive heart failure can be examined by using M-mode or two-dimensional echocardiography. These two types of ultrasound can be extremely helpful for excluding a number of conditions that might be missed on other tests.

Echocardiography is an excellent way to study patients who have suspected pericardial effusion. Normally, there are echoes off the two layers of pericardium. When an effusion is present, a relatively echo-free space occurs between the epicardium and pericardium (Chung, 1986).

Three major types of ultrasound imaging are available today: M-mode, two-dimensional, and Doppler. M-mode and two-dimensional echocardiography provide dynamic images of the heart, and Doppler echocardiography records the blood flow within arteries and veins. When two-dimensional and Doppler echocardiography are combined, the technique is called color flow mapping.

M-mode echocardiography produces single-frame pictures of the aortic and mitral valves and of the left ventricle. It can be used to assess left ventricular volume, ejection fraction, and filling and ejection rates.

Two-dimensional echocardiography looks at the heart in two dimensions and while the organ is moving. With this method, the examiner can see all four heart valves and all four heart chambers. Valvular vegetations and ventricular function can be evaluated better with this method than with the M-mode technique. Recordings are made that can be displayed on a movie film or videotape (Fulkerson, 1985).

Doppler ultrasound detects blood flow velocity. Measurement of blood velocity in the ascending aorta gives information about left ventricular function. Blood velocity in the pulmonary artery gives information about right ventricular function and pulmonary vascular resistance. Doppler studies also can measure pressure gradients across the heart valves (Sokolow et al., 1990).

Often Doppler ultrasound is combined with two-dimensional echocardiography to study structure and function together. This color mapping can be done because the color is proportional to the velocity of blood flow. The examiner is able to see valve lesions and determine flow problems at the same time, thus detecting stenosis or regurgitation (Sokolow et al., 1990).

Echocardiographic results are limited by the physical characteristics of the patient and the experience and skill of the examiner. Persons who have large, thick chest walls and small hearts, and those who have chest deformities are difficult to examine. Proper direction of the transducer is important to avoid the lungs and bony thorax.

Despite these limitations, echocardiography is an excellent way to study left ventricular volume, ejection fraction, wall motion, contractility, valve function, shunting, and effusions. It is noninvasive and avoids the damaging effects of x-rays.

Preparation of the patient. Although no physiologic preparation is needed for echocardiography, patients need basic explanations of the testing procedure. They should know that the test is noninvasive and causes no discomfort. They may be positioned on their sides to make it easier for the examiner to direct the transducer toward cardiac structures. If the Doppler technique is used, patients hear the swishing sound of blood flow, and they need to know that this is normal. The examination takes about 30 min.

DIGITAL SUBTRACTION ANGIOGRAPHY

Digital subtraction angiography is a computerized method that does not require cardiac catheterization and is used to evaluate the function of the left side of the heart. Contrast material is injected into the right side of the heart, and images are obtained as the material goes through the heart. Only structures containing contrast material appear, without interference from other structures. After a second image is obtained, the computer subtracts the previous image. This subtraction of the images that are the same in both pictures leaves only the different area showing.

Image gating coordinates images with certain aspects of the cardiac cycle, thus eliminating some of the motion problems. Although the images are not as clear as those obtained with coronary angiography, the examiner can see the major blood vessels and cardiac chambers and can calculate ejection fraction and evaluate wall motion. Imaging problems occur if the chamber is enlarged or valvular regurgitation occurs, which could disperse the contrast agent, making it less concentrated in the area being viewed.

Patients must lie still and hold their breath during imaging (about 20–30 sec). They also must not swallow so that they do not move other structures that might obscure the image. These requirements are difficult for very sick patients and may limit the use of this technique.

Complications. Two major types of complications can occur with angiocardiography, those caused by mechanical trauma from the catheter and the force of the injected stream of contrast material and those due to the pharmacologic effects of the contrast material. The heart may be perforated or the contrast medium may be injected into the myocardium. Usually, perforation of a ventricle produces no serious side effects. Perforation of the atrium is a more serious complication of catheterization. The thinner atrial walls cannot seal off the puncture site as well as the ventricular wall can, and more blood usually pours out into the pericardium during atrial perforation. The bleeding often stops spontaneously, and it is not necessary to rush the patient to surgery once bleeding is discovered. The catheter should be removed and the patient's vital signs carefully monitored. If blood has accumulated in the pericardium, this can usually be measured by using echocardiography or computed tomography.

COMPUTED TOMOGRAPHY

Computed tomography (CT) is expensive, uses significant amounts of ionizing radiation, and has some difficulty imaging moving structures. Yet it is being used more often in some centers to determine the patency of aortocoronary bypass grafts, detect anterior MI, outline aortic dissections, show intracardiac tumors or thrombi, and show calcifications in the coronary vessels or pericardium. CT scanning distinguishes differences in density between various tissues and fluids. Radiopaque contrast material is used to enhance those differences. Patients must lie still and hold their breath during the few seconds of scanning (Sokolow et al., 1990).

NUCLEAR IMAGING

Nuclear imaging is done by injecting specially prepared radioactive materials that can be detected in the bloodstream or tissues by a gamma camera. This technique can be used for many body systems. In the cardiovascular system, we are referring to myocardial imaging. This imaging can be done to assess perfusion and infarction and to look at the structure and the functional activity of the heart.

As discussed in the section on the use of radionuclides during stress testing, thallium can be used to assess perfusion of the heart. Thallium-201 is injected intravenously, and scanning of the heart is started 5–10 min after the injection. Normally, the myocardium picks up the thallium. Areas of poor perfusion appear dark on the scan ("cold spots"). If an abnormality appears, the scan is repeated in 3–24 hr. If reperfusion has occurred, the earlier problem was ischemia. If the scan remains unchanged, the earlier problem was infarcted muscle. This is also a useful test for assessing myocardial perfusion before and after coronary bypass grafting.

Myocardial imaging can be done to detect infarcted areas. The material used in this situation is technetium-^{99m}–Tc labeled pyrophosphate that is injected intravenously. Two hours after the injection, the scanning is done with the gamma camera. Concentration of ^{99m}Tc in infarcted muscle begins 10–12 hr after infarction peaks at 72 hr, and lasts about a week. In patients who have delayed seeking medical attention after having an MI, the injury can be diagnosed by using ^{99m}Tc, even after enzyme and ECG changes have normalized. The scan gives a good indication of the extent of the infarction (Sokolow et al., 1990).

Radionuclide angiography is a third type of nuclear imaging test. In the first-pass procedure, sodium pertechnetate, another technetium compound, is injected intravenously, and scanning is done as the agent flows through the heart, outlining the heart chambers. This is a particularly good way to assess right ventricular ejection fraction. In the gated equilibrium technique, ^{99m}Tc-labeled red blood cells are injected and allowed to equilibrate with the blood volume. Scanning can begin in 5-10 min and can be done up to 6 hr after injection. "Gated" means that imaging is restricted to certain times in the cardiac cycle (determined by the ECG). These images are stored and then averaged to give a summary picture. Ejection fraction can be calculated and wall motion problems can be detected by using this technique. The gated study can be used during exercise, but the patient's movement results in less clear images.

Positive emission tomography is a relatively new and expensive method of assessing the metabolic processes of the heart. A radionuclider, ^{18}F-2-fluoro-2-deoxyglucose, is injected, and its uptake by cardiac tissue followed. The agent has such a short half-life that a cyclotron must be present in the building in which the study is being performed. Uptake of the radionuclide indicates areas of metabolism and therefore areas of viable heart tissue. The technique is used to distinguish between old and new MIs and between ischemic, but viable, and dead myocardium. Because of its expense, the need for a cyclotron, and differences in results between patients who have been fed and those who have fasted, this test is not often used (Sokolow et al., 1990).

A similar test, which is less expensive and also less accurate, is single-photon emission computed tomography. This test uses conventional radionuclides, ^{99m}Tc and ^{201}TI, and does not require a cyclotron. The quality of this test result is between the qualities of the results of positron emission tomography and conventional CT scans (Sokolow et al., 1990).

MAGNETIC RESONANCE IMAGING

Magnetic resonance imaging (MRI) is a new diagnostic tool for assessing cardiovascular disease. It was used originally to detect masses in the chest, abdomen, head, and neck. Now it is a valuable technique for diagnosing aortic aneurysm and for distinguishing between constrictive pericarditis and restrictive cardiomyopathy. It is also useful in measuring ejection fraction, ventricular wall motion, and blood flow in the heart and great vessels.

MRI uses a strong magnetic field to pull information from body cells. The nuclei of atoms in body cells have magnetic properties and spin around their axes like tops. When a magnetic force is applied, the nuclei spin into a different alignment, and when the force is removed, they relax again. This changing of position is detected as energy signals and is measurable. The signals from various tissues differ mostly because of differences in water content. "Wet" tissues produce more signals than "dry" tissues do.

The advantages of MRI include superior contrast of soft tissues, elimination of exposure to x-rays, acquisition of images on multiple planes that would be obscured by bone on CT scans or radiographs, noninvasiveness, and no requirement for contrast material. As good as MRI sounds, it also has some disadvantages. The patient must lie still for several minutes during the imaging, a requirement that can be difficult for someone who has back problems or difficulty breathing. It is contraindicated for patients who have implanted metal objects such as pacemakers, vascular clips, metal heart valves, prosthetic joints, or insulin pumps. These objects can become magnetized, causing them to move or function abnormally. The imager cannot accommodate obese people or those who are physiologically unstable and require life support equipment. MRI is an expensive diagnostic test and usually is reserved for those in whom results of other diagnostic tests were inconclusive.

Preparation of the patient. Physical preparation is minimal for this test. Patients do not need to be without food, water, or medications unless the abdomen is being scanned. They should use the bathroom before imaging begins, because the entire procedure may last 1.5 hr. They should remove metal clips; eyeglasses; hearing aids; dentures; watches; and clothing with metal zippers, buttons, or other fasteners. They should be sure they do not have any cards with magnetic stripes in their pockets. Psychologically, patients must be prepared for the closed environment, the need to lie still, and the thumping noise from the machine. They will be relieved to know that they will not receive injections or feel pain from the test other than the discomfort of lying still.

CARDIAC CATHETERIZATION/ CORONARY ANGIOGRAPHY

The term cardiac catheterization frequently is used to mean both cardiac catheterization and coronary angiography. To the layperson, the two procedures appear to be the same: tubes are threaded through blood vessels to examine problems in the heart. Both procedures are done with local anesthesia in the cardiac catheterization laboratory and are done by the same health team. The patient feels the same after each procedure and requires nearly the same care. However, these procedures are different.

In a cardiac catheterization, the catheters are threaded up a major vein (femoral vein entered percutaneously or brachial vein entered via a cutdown) into the right side of the heart and as far as the pulmonary artery. Contrast material can be injected into the right atrium to observe blood flow through the heart, including flow through abnormal openings (atrial septal defects and ventricular septal defects), impaired forward flow (valvular stenosis), or backward flow (valvular regurgitation). Blood samples are analyzed for oxygen content to evaluate abnormal septal openings that allow oxygenated blood from the left side of the heart to mix with deoxygenated blood from the right side of the heart. Pressures are measured in the right atrium, right ventricle, and pulmonary artery to evaluate valvular dysfunctions, pulmonary hypertension, and left-sided heart problems reflected back toward the pulmonary artery. If the patient will be cared

for in the intensive care unit (ICU), the pulmonary artery catheter may be left indwelling for several days for repeated measurements of right atrial, pulmonary artery, and pulmonary capillary wedge pressure.

With coronary angiography, a major artery is entered either percutaneously (femoral artery) or via a cutdown (brachial artery), and the catheter is passed retrogradely up the aorta and into the left ventricle. When the catheter is in the ventricle, pressures are recorded, and then the catheter is pulled back into the aorta for more pressure readings to assess the pressure gradient between the two chambers. A second catheter carries a contrast medium into the left ventricle, which helps in the assessment of volumes, regional wall motion, and ejection fraction. The catheter then is pulled back to the aorta where special catheters are directed down right and left coronary arteries. Contrast material injected down the coronary catheters helps the examiner visualize the coronary arteries and obstructions to blood flow. Coronary angiography is commonly recorded on film for later viewing and assessment.

Preparation of the Patient. Knowledge of why the test is being done will help you provide explanations to the patient and allay his or her fears. Assess the patient's allergies, especially those to iodine, povidone-iodine (Betadine), and shellfish, because the contrast material is iodine based. Know the patient's usual medications and if the physician wants them held or given on schedule. Assess and mark peripheral pulses for comparison after the procedure.

The procedure is invasive, so the patient must give informed consent. The physician should explain the indications for the procedure, the steps in the procedure, and potential complications. Frequently, the nurse will need to reexplain aspects of the procedure and answer the patient's questions. Standardized teaching booklets and videos are helpful. In addition to basic procedural information, patients should know that they will be on a movable table; will be covered with sterile sheets, which they should not touch; and will be conscious throughout the testing. They will have ECG monitoring leads on and one or more intravenous lines, and a lot of complex equipment will be present in the room. Health team personnel will talk among themselves using unfamiliar words, but they will give directions to the patient by addressing him or her by name. Patients should expect to feel a hot flash and experience a salty taste when the contrast material is injected. However, if they feel any pain during the procedure, they should tell the physician or nurse immediately.

Postprocedure care. The most important postprocedure assessments are concerned with circulation to the extremity used for the catheterization and to the heart. Check the catheter insertion site and pulses distal to it each time you record the patient's vital signs. Note and report to the physician overt bleeding, formation of hematomas, swelling of the thigh, and loss of pulse. Note also temperature of the involved extremity, sensation, and capillary filling. Assessment usually also includes monitoring vital signs every 15 min for four times, then every 30–60 min for four times, and then every 4 hr. Hypotension, tachycardia, rhythm irregularities, and chest pain should be reported to the physician immediately in addition to abnormal findings. The patient usually is ordered to drink 2–3L of fluid during the first 6–8 hr after the procedure to flush the contrast material out of the body. Patients unable to drink adequately need intravenous fluid therapy. Patients need to talk about the experience. Once the physician has explained the findings and treatment options, they may need further clarification of what they have learned. Be careful to listen and clarify, and encourage patients to discuss concerns with their cardiologist.

OTHER INVASIVE STUDIES

Other invasive studies that are done include measurements of coronary blood velocity and electrophysiologic studies. For measurements of coronary blood flow, small catheters with transducers are inserted into the coronary arteries. Papaverine (12 mg) is given through the coronary arteries. Coronary flow is expected to increase four to five times. Failure to increase flow suggests coronary disease.

Electrophysiologic studies are done for patients who have intractable dysrhythmias unrelieved by usual medications or who have experienced near sudden death. The conduction system as it passes through the interventricular septum can be studied. Patients who need adjustment in medication to suppress serious ventricular dysrhythmias may have electrophysioligic testing. The dysrhythmia is induced in the controlled setting of the catheterization laboratory where it can be terminated by overdrive pacing or defibrillation if medications do not work. This is safer than the trial-and-error method of trying a drug and waiting to see if the patient experiences a near sudden death again, perhaps in an area without appropriate life support readily available (Sokolow et al., 1990).

The patient about to have electrophysiologic testing may be understandably anxious about being put purposefully into a life-threatening rhythm. Encourage verbalization of these feelings, and reinforce the concept that the purpose of the test is to prevent the development of these rhythms in the uncontrolled settings of daily life where they might be fatal. Printed teaching materials and visits from patients who have had electrophysiologic testing are helpful in providing realistic information for these patients.

TABLE 10
Summary of Diagnostic Tests for Cardiac Disease

Test	Uses
Chest radiography	Assess size and shape of heart Assess pulmonary congestion
Electrocardiography	Assess electrical activity of the heart Detect myocardial infarction (MI), enlargement, electrical disturbances, and ischemia Monitor drug effects
Exercise tests	Detect mechanical abnormalities Test functional capacity of cardiac patients Estimate cardiac prognosis Test healthy persons for activities that demand high levels of physical activity
Radionuclide stress test	Assess myocardial perfusion and ventricular function
Echocardiography	Evaluate left ventricular function Show pericardial effusion Examine heart valves
Digital subtraction angiography	Calculate ejection fraction Evaluate wall motion
Computed tomography (CT)	See patency of aortocoronary grafts Detect anterior MI, aortic dissections, intracardiac tumors or thrombi, and calcification in coronary arteries or pericardium
Nuclear imaging	Assess myocardial perfusion
Thallium	Detect infarcted muscle
Technetium pyrophosphate	Good for patients who come to the hospital late in the infarction
Sodium pertechnetate	Assess ejection fraction
Technetium-tagged erythrocytes	Assess ejection fraction and wall motion
Positron emission tomography (PET)	Distinguish between viable and dead myocardium (requires a cyclotron and is costly)
Single-photon emission computed tomography	Is less expensive, but less accurate than PET
Magnetic resonance imaging (MRI)	Visualize aortic aneurysm Distinguish constrictive pericarditis from restrictive cardiomyopathy Assess ejection fraction and wall motion
Cardiac catheterization	Detect abnormal heart valves, septal defects, abnormal heart and lung pressures
Coronary angiography	Visualize coronary blood flow and obstructions
Coronary blood velocity measurements	Measure blood flow and ability of coronary arteries to increase flow
Electrophysiologic studies	Locate source of intractable dysrhythmias and determine effective treatments

COMPLICATIONS OF INVASIVE STUDIES

Invasive studies that require the introduction of mechanical instruments into the heart and blood vessels are associated with many potential complications. The blood vessels can be damaged by trauma, causing vessel spasm, dissections, or fistulas. Bleeding or emboli at catheter insertion sites are common complications. The previously discussed postprocedure assessments to detect circulatory problems can help detect problems early for rapid intervention. Emergency surgery to correct vascular problems may be needed (Sokolow et al., 1990).

Dysrhythmias may occur because of mechanical stimulation by catheters, because of vasovagal responses, or because of irritation caused by contrast media. The presence of catheters in the right atrium of a patient who has atrial septal defects or mitral valve disease may precipitate atrial dysrhythmias. The presence of catheters in the right ventricle may cause PVCs, ventricular tachycardia, or ventricular fibrillation. When catheters are removed, the patient may have a vasovagal response with decreasing blood pressure, heart rate, and level of consciousness. For these reasons, it is important to have emergency medication and a defibrillator readily available during and immediately after these procedures (Sokolow et al., 1990).

In addition to dysrhythmias, the contrast medium can cause fluid imbalances. It is hyperosmotic and increases blood volume. Patients with healthy kidneys excrete the medium in the urine and could become hypovolemic if their fluid intake is inadequate. If patients are unable to excrete the fluid, pulmonary edema may develop. Patients with known renal failure are generally scheduled for hemodialysis immediately after the procedure.

A final complication to consider concerns the health team. Physicians and nurses are exposed to significant amounts of radiation and blood during these invasive studies. They need to wear protective lead aprons, radiation badges, gloves, goggles, and other protective clothing to avoid exposure.

CHAPTER 5

Questions 39–51

39. A chest radiograph can be used to detect which of the following?

    a. Pulmonary congestion

    b. Valvular stenosis

    c. Decreased ejection fraction

    d. Pulmonary emboli

40. Patients who are having continuous ECG monitoring need to know which of the following?

    a. They should hold still throughout the monitoring.

    b. They may feel tiny electric shocks from time to time.

    c. Any discomfort they are having will show up on the monitor.

    d. Monitor alarms do not necessarily mean a serious problem.

41. One purpose of a treadmill stress test is to:

    a. Diagnose MI

    b. Assess myocardial ischemia with activity

    c. Test physical endurance of patients with severe aortic stenosis

    d. Help obese patients lose weight to decrease risk of coronary disease

42. People who should not undergo low-level ECG stress tests include:

    a. Those with mild hypertension

    b. Those with serious cardiac arrhythmias

    c. Diabetic patient's

    d. Obese patients

43. Exercise stress testing can be continued as long as:

    a. The heart rate remains the same

    b. The blood pressure remains the same

    c. The patient does not complain of chest pain, marked fatigue, or syncope

    d. There are no heart arrhythmias

44. Dipyridamole thallium stress testing might be more beneficial than regular thallium stress testing for which of the following persons?

    a. Patient with an amputation of the right leg

    b. Healthy persons being tested for an insurance physical

    c. Patient in acute congestive heart failure

    d. Patient who has had an MI

45. In preparing patients for echocardiography, the nurse tells them which of the following?

    a. They will be rolled into a large machine with an echo chamber.

    b. They will need to wear earplugs to minimize the echo sound.

    c. The test will cause a feeling of pressure as the sound waves hit tissues.

    d. Sound waves will be bounced painlessly off the heart to give a picture of it.

46. One purpose of nuclear imaging is to:

    a. Measure cardiac output

    b. Detect an MI as it is occurring

    c. Assess valvular stenosis or regurgitation

    d. Assess myocardial perfusion before and after coronary bypass grafting

47. One purpose of magnetic resonance imaging is to:

    a. Differentiate between constrictive pericarditis and restrictive cardiomyopathy

    b. Diagnose MI

    c. Visualize broken ribs

    d. Detect rhythm abnormalities

48. After cardiac catheterization, the pulmonary artery catheter may be left in place to measure:

    a. Right ventricular pressure

    b. Pulmonary capillary wedge pressure

    c. Arterial blood pressure

    d. Ejection fraction

49. In coronary angiography, what is the physician studying?

    a. Heart valves

    b. Lung tissue

    c. Coronary arteries

    d. Septal defects

50. Patients may have electrophysiologic studies for which of the following reasons?

    a. Unifocal PVCs

    b. Atrial fibrillation

    c. Chest pain associated with physical activity

    d. Ventricular dysrhythmias unresponsive to usual medications

51. A finding after an invasive procedure that requires the immediate attention of a physician is:

    a. Increased urine output

    b. Occasional appearance of PVCs

    c. Formation of a hematoma at the catheterization site

    d. Pulses distal to the catheterization site

CHAPTER 6

PSYCHOSOCIAL ASPECTS OF CARDIOVASCULAR DISEASE

CHAPTER OBJECTIVE

After studying this chapter, the reader will be able to recognize common psychological responses to acute cardiac illness and those that occur in recovery phases.

LEARNING OBJECTIVES

After studying this chapter, the reader will be able to

1. Name at least two common responses to signs and symptoms of heart disease.

2. Differentiate between normal and abnormal psychological responses to acute cardiac illnesses.

3. State three characteristics of near-death experiences.

4. State two common family responses to acute illness of a family member.

5. Name three behaviors seen in patients in the recovery phase of cardiac illness.

INTRODUCTION

Persons at risk for CHD share may common physiologic and psychosocial behavior traits. No one trait causes CHD, but the combination of traits increases the likelihood of the disease developing. Some traits cannot be changed, but most can be modified to decrease the risk of CHD. Chapters 1–3 discuss many risk factors and barriers to change. This chapter briefly reviews psychological risk factors. You will go beyond pre-CHD assessment to learning about common responses of patients and their families to critical cardiac illnesses. You will then follow the recovering patient into discharge and rehabilitation phases.

BEHAVIORS BEFORE THE ILLNESS

In addition to the physiologic risk factors for CHD, some psychological behaviors are common in persons in whom CHD develops. Friedman and Rosenman (1974) have called this type A behavior or coronary-prone behavior. They contrast this behavior with type B behavior. In reality, few persons are purely type A or type B. Most have combinations of behavior styles, but tend to lean one way or the other. Some behaviors are learned while the person is growing up; some develop later. None are so much a part of the personality that they cannot be changed. However, change can be difficult and requires the patient's commitment to be successful.

Type A behaviors typically occur in achievement-oriented persons who work with great intensity, aggression, and urgency to accomplish tasks. These persons tend to struggle to fit more and more into less and less time. A type A person is always rushed, is impatient while waiting, and has difficulty letting others finish their thoughts or sentences. Type A persons expect others to share this intensity and to make the same commitments. The feeling of time urgency makes it difficult for type A persons to take time to be creative and leads them into stereotyped behavior in which they cannot accept change. This achievement orientation is not limited to work; it extends into family relationships and the few outside activities that type A persons permit themselves. They may demand high achievement from their children in school or expect to be always on the winning team or to own the best car or home.

A nurse who works with type A persons needs to understand their intense behavior patterns. Recognizing stress as a CHD risk factor is important. Telling patients to "decrease stress" will be futile. Patients must really believe that a stress reaction is harmful before they will attempt to change their behavior. Patients who have chest pain during an intense business meeting may be able to correlate stress with heart disease. Patients may believe that they are at risk if others in their peer group, who share the same lifestyles, have heart attacks or must have cardiac surgery. Patients who have asymptomatic CHD will be the hardest to convince.

Patients who do relate their stress reactions to heart disease may have one or more responses. These who perceive heart disease as a realistic threat to their lives may be motivated to make lifestyle changes. Changes frequently are temporary because patients revert to their previous coping styles. Denial of illness and total restrictions in activity are opposite ways persons use to cope with a threat to their body image. A broken leg would slow down physical activity, but a diseased heart cannot be seen and therefore can be denied. Others are frightened by this threat, and they restrict all activity, becoming "cardiac invalids." Threats to self-image (the way a person sees himself or herself in relation to social and work roles) may make a person feel changed in an indescribable way. A patient may feel that he or she is no longer a competent provider or spouse, is not the same dynamic leader at work, or is useless.

BEHAVIORS DURING THE ACUTE ILLNESS

Shock and disbelief. During the acute phase of cardiac illness, patients generally experience a normal grief response. The most common response to MI is denial. Patients have a host of explanations for their symptoms—indigestion, pulled muscle, toothache, and so forth. They rationalize their signs and symptoms by saying, "This cannot be happening to me. I just had a complete physical," or "I don't think my heart is the problem. Let me out of here." It is important that lay persons be aware of this reaction and act quickly to obtain needed medical help. In the hospital setting, nurses need to know how the patient describes the symptoms: "pressure," "indigestion," "arm pain," or "chest pain." A patient who is experiencing intense substernal pressure may give a negative response to a question about chest pain and thus delay treatment. While denying the severity of the illness, the patient also experiences fear, thinking, What is happening to me? Am I dying? This stage of shock and disbelief lasts a few minutes to a few days.

During the period of denial, it is important that the nurse not try to strip away this defense mechanism. Denial in the first hours and days of illness protects the patient from anxiety and fear. Anxiety and fear will increase the release of catecholamines, increasing the myocardial workload of an already compromised heart and thus promoting further damage to the heart. Arguing with a patient in denial also increases the release of catecholamines and cardiac work. Nursing actions need to support reality but not force it on the patient. Patients who will not believe that their heart is the problem and who want to be released from the ICU can be told, "I know it's hard to believe your heart could be the problem. Just to be sure, we need to keep you here for a few days to check blood tests and ECGs, which will give us the answer. How can I make your time here more comfortable?" Fear during this stage can be minimized with calm, truthful explanations and frequent bedside interactions. Sedative medications may be useful also, but they never should be used in place of interpersonal communication.

Developing awareness. When patients realize that something is wrong with their hearts, they are developing awareness. In this stage, they move in and out of anger, bargaining, and depression. Anger may be directed at themselves or others, with comments such as, "I did what my doctor said, but I still had a heart attack. What kind of doctor is he?" or "Why didn't I stop smoking earlier?" or "You don't let me sleep. No wonder I'm sick!" Bargaining usually is done with a higher power or authority. It is not unusual to hear a patient say, "If I only live through this, I'll go to church regularly," or "If I get better, I'll stop smoking." Depression is common 3–5 days after an MI (Thelan, Davie, & Viden, 1990). This is a time when the patients' signs and symptoms usually have resolved, and their focus turns to what has happened to them and how it will affect their lives. Feelings of powerlessness and low self-esteem are common: "I cannot do anything now. What good am I as a husband?"

As patients enter the period of developing awareness, they may often lash out in anger. Remember that many MI patients are type A personalities who cope with stress by trying to control the situation and who are impatient with anything outside their usual activities. Anger may be expressed in words or in actions (e.g., pulling off leads, climbing over side rails, or refusing treatments). The nurse should avoid arguing with patients but should set limits to protect patients from harming themselves or others. Sometimes

giving patients more control over their situation decreases anger and increases compliance.

Bargaining may be done with a higher power, and patients may wish to see a clergy member. Bargains with physicians and nurses are usually long-term proposals (e.g., "I'll quit smoking if I live through this") and need little intervention other than active listening. Short-term "deals" (e.g., "I'll take my medicine if I can walk to the bathroom") should be addressed on an individual basis.

Depression is a source of concern to family members who now see the patient improving physically and cannot understand the patient's failure to feel positive. It is important to explain to both the patient and the family that this is a normal stage of recovery. To help move patients through depression, increase their activity as soon as possible. Use a firm, kind approach to maintain the patient's self-respect as you get the patient up and bathed. Specific directions such as "Walk to the next doorway and back three times each day" are more helpful than "Gradually increase your activity." Depression that lasts longer than 1 week may require psychiatric assessment.

ICU psychosis. ICU psychosis may occur in some patients within 2–5 days of their admission to the unit. Because the patients' usual behaviors and usual state of health are not known to the ICU staff, some of the subtle behavioral changes that precede the more obvious psychosis may be missed. Characteristics of ICU psychosis are impaired intellectual function, difficulty in judging reality, and an altered emotional state in a high-stress situation. Behavioral manifestations may include the following:

- Having auditory and visual hallucinations (hearing and seeing things not present)

- Misinterpreting stimuli (confusion about health personnel in scrub suits, who are interpreted as businesspersons inappropriately attired in pajamas)

- Talking with people not present (family, spirits)

- Having feelings of persecution, especially related to painful procedures (e.g., suctioning, intravenous procedures, moving into a CT scanner)

- Pulling at tubes and wires and possibly causing harm to self

- Trying to get away from perceived danger by climbing out of bed

Factors that promote ICU psychosis include the following:

- Disturbed sleep cycles

- Absence of a day-night cycle

- Frequent contact with the many staff members for care

- Overhearing staff members on rounds talk about the patients

- Proximity of other patients with their inherent odors, noises, and activities

- Multiple pieces of equipment within the line of vision

- Meaningless noises of machines

- Lack of usual sensory stimulation

- Sedation, which blurs consciousness

- History of psychiatric illness or of drug or alcohol abuse

- Prolonged cardiopulmonary bypass

Treatment of ICU psychosis. If admission to an ICU is anticipated (as occurs with patients who have cardiac surgery), preoperative teaching can help minimize the confusion. Patients need to know that confusion and frightening dreams are common and do not indicate a psychiatric problem. They should be encouraged to discuss their fears before the operation and to share their feelings afterward. Unplanned admission to the ICU adds another stressor for the patient.

To minimize ICU psychosis, decrease unnecessary stimuli. Move equipment out of the patient's line of vision. Turn off lights at night. Keep the patient oriented to the environment, ICU personnel, time, and current events. Explain all procedures before doing them. Be truthful about uncomfortable procedures. Involve the family in the patient's care if they desire. Simple activities such as applying a cool cloth to the patient's head can be comforting to both the patient and the family (Guzzelta & Dossey, 1984).

If ICU psychosis does occur, continue orientation activities. Be very simple and concrete in explanations. Do not agree with hallucinations, but do not belittle the patient. Statements such as the following do not take away the patient's self-respect, yet they promote reality orientation: "I do not see those dogs that you see. I think they will go away as you get healthier." Support family members who may be frightened by the patient's bizarre behavior. Assure them that this is a temporary state and that it will pass.

Fortunately, ICU psychosis frequently passes after 24–48 hr on the regular nursing unit. Some confusion may take several days to resolve. Many patients do not remember any of the specific details of this period and need not be reminded. Patients' behaviors may be very uncharacteristic and an unnecessary source of embarrassment for them.

Near-death experiences. The near-death experience is a psychological phenomenon of persons who come close to death. Some studies suggest that up to 50% of persons who come very close to death may have this experience. Many persons who have had a near-death experience are afraid to discuss it, thinking that they will be considered crazy. Others do not discuss it until many years after the experience.

Regardless of the person's age, sex, culture, religion, education, social class, or occupation, all near-death experiences have many things in common:

- Separation from the body occurs. Persons can relate what actually happened to them during the time they were out of their bodies, describe people never seen before or since, and tell how they felt as the health team worked to save their lives (some hoped not to be saved, others hoped the resuscitation would be successful).

- Moving through a dark tunnel or space or through a fog is common. Many see a bright light on the other side that is associated with peace, love, and serenity.

- Many meet deceased relatives or friends, some of whom they may have had no knowledge of before the experience.

- Some meet a religious figure appropriate to their culture. This is not restricted to believers; it also occurs with atheists.

- Persons see their lives pass before them or see significant people in their lives.

- Usually a sense of calm and relief from pain occur.

- Despite the pleasantness of the experience and the anticipation of pain on return, the persons understand a need to return to the body and do so.

- After the experience, persons have a sense of knowing about love and truth that they did not have before, and frequently they make lifestyle changes to promote this love.

Caring for a patient who has had a near-death experience requires sensitivity and patience. Even before you realize that a patient has had such an experience, you can help such patients by talking to them to keep them oriented about things going on during the period of unconsciousness. Patients may be afraid to come right out and explain their experience for fear of being ridiculed. You can say that many persons who have been through a crisis like this have unusual experiences and leave an open-ended invitation for patients to talk about their own feelings. It is important not to label near-death experiences as drug reactions or psychopathologic responses. Do not prod the patients; let them tell about their experience at their own pace. Reassure them that others have had similar experiences and refer them to support groups as needed (Corcoran, 1988).

Transfer anxiety. The critically ill patient becomes dependent on the care of one or more nurses. Such patients are told that they are seriously ill, that they need total rest, that they need to let others care for them. If the moment of transfer from the ICU comes suddenly, the patient may be fearful that he or she is being abandoned. This type of anxiety also can occur as care is transferred from one nurse to another within the ICU setting (Holloway, 1988).

Transfer out of the ICU should be treated as a graduation or promotion to be eagerly anticipated rather than as a feeling of being dumped out for another patient's admission. In order to minimize transfer anxiety, it is important to prepare patients for the move. Help them track their progress, for example, progressive ambulation, less intravenous medication to control chest pain, resolution of dysrhythmias, and healing of wounds. Give them progressively more responsibility for self-care. For example, although a nurse could do the job more quickly, allow patients to bathe themselves to provide more independence and self-confidence. Inform patients of the expected length of stay in the ICU and where they will be cared for next. At the time of transfer, introduce the patient to the new nurse (also applicable to shift-to-shift transfer within the ICU). This helps patients see that both nurses are part of the team and that care will be continued. If you promise to visit a patient after the transfer, keep your promise.

Sometimes patients are transferred suddenly because a more critically ill patient is admitted. This should be avoided if possible, because patients may not feel ready to leave the ICU. If possible, visit suddenly transferred patients soon after the transfer to assure them of your interest in their welfare and your coordination of their care with their new nurses.

EMOTIONAL RESPONSE TO HEART SURGERY

Deciding to have surgery. Deciding to have surgery is one of the biggest decisions many persons make in a lifetime. The heart, the symbol of life, love, and courage, will be stopped, handled, cut, and sewn. No guarantee can be given that the operation will be successful or even that it will not be harmful. The patient looks forward to pain, prolonged recovery, financial expense, and possibly death.

Several factors can help prospective patients and their families. Patients who see the surgery as giving them a new lease on life will approach the procedure positively. Patients who see the benefits of surgery outweighing the risks will probably consent to the procedure.

In one survey, patients were quite concerned with the need for psychological support. Several received no support from family physicians, cardiologists, or surgeons (Borders, 1985, 1986). Patients may have preconceived ideas about heart surgery from the positive and negative experiences of friends, from popular magazines and television programs, from fellow patients, or from their own previous hospital experiences. They may have received medical information they did not understand. They may have unique concerns about family life, work, and finances. Whenever possible, a group approach to preoperative teaching is useful to help patients share common concerns and develop a support group; such an approach is also economical and time efficient for hospitals.

Postoperative phase. A patient may awaken after surgery feeling confused. The patient has lost a big block of time while under anesthesia and awakens multiple invasive lines. Although patients may appear to be awake, several hours may pass before they are fully awake. If they have had good preoperative instructions, a simple explanation of what is being done usually sets their minds at ease. If the surgery was emergent and no preoperative teaching was possible, the patient will need frequent explanations of care and restrictions.

Pain is usually a major postoperative concern. Many patients have no pain when still and only mild pain with activity. Others have significant pain while at rest and excruciating incisional chest pain with coughing and incisional leg pain with walking. The nurse should be aware of these variations in pain response and should medicate patients adequately according to their needs. Patients who are pain-free are more relaxed and more cooperate during treatments.

After the initial realization that they have survived surgery and made it through 2 days of clinical progress, patients often have a period of depression. This is similar to the depression seen in patients 3–4 days after an MI. During this stage, patients cry easily, feel sicker, and have memory lapses. Patients who have been forewarned of this reaction usually have a less intense depression.

Going home. Going home is a major milestone after heart surgery, but the joy is tempered by anxiety at leaving the security of the hospital. As with the transfer anxiety that occurs when moving from ICU to step-down or ward care, this anxiety can be minimized by good preparation, written instructions, and a telephone number to call for questions. Some hospitals have a nurse make a follow-up call to the patient's home the day after discharge to help ease the transition or have a home health nurse visit the home.

THE FAMILY'S RESPONSE TO ILLNESS

Families are an integral part of the patient's life and need to be considered when care is planned. The acute physiologic needs of the patient are always of prime importance. Ideally, the patient's nurse will be able to care for the family too. However, many times the staffing demands of the unit do not provide for an extended time with families. In this situation, a social worker or a member of the clergy may be designated for family support. This should not be left for whoever is available; it should be a designated assignment for some member of the health care team.

When patients are critically ill, their families may be isolated from them for extended periods. Events may have evolved rapidly, leaving family members disoriented and afraid that their loved one may die. Depending on life circumstances and usual coping behaviors, family members may feel anger at the patient or the health care team for the illness, guilt that they did not push the patient to treatment earlier, or depression and grief.

Family members react to these stressors in varied ways. They may minimize the illness to decrease the threat it imposes. Some intellectualize the illness by focusing on the technical aspects of care and blocking out emotional responses. Some repeat information received or the sequence of events as if to convince themselves of their appropriate response. One or more family members may be strong and supportive for other members. Many want to remain close to the patient, either at the bedside or in a nearby waiting room (Kleinpell, 1991).

Nurses should be aware of the family's needs. Nursing research studies have determined needs of families of critically ill patients. Overall, the top one has been the need to have hope. The studies also have shown that frequently nurses do not rank family needs in the same order as families do.

Family members should be encouraged to talk with the nurse, social worker, or clergy as well as among themselves. Verbalizing fears and needs is usually more helpful than keeping silent. Provide privacy during brief family visits in the ICU. Encourage hugs, kisses, or other signs of affection if desired. Make yourself available to a designated family member who calls to get a report on the patient's condition. Convey all messages to the patient. This kind of tie to the family at home can be very therapeutic.

Once the critical illness is over and the patient is moved out of ICU, families may be forgotten. Without frequent updates and progress reports, family members imagine all sorts of complications occurring. Keep patients and families aware of progress to decrease unnecessary anxiety and to prepare a smooth transition to discharge from the hospital.

Homecoming for any cardiac patient may be met with a variety of emotions. The spouse may harbor suppressed anger at the patient for being ill. The spouse may feel of guilty if the illness occurred during sexual relations or when the patient was doing work for the spouse. Spouses frequently overprotect the patient both as an expression of love and concern and out of fear that something will go wrong. Open communication in the hospital and at home is the key to minimizing homecoming anxiety (Rankin, 1992).

RECOVERY BEHAVIORS

Recovery is a prolonged period that begins with discharge from the hospital and lasts for the rest of the patient's life. It starts when patients return to their homes. Patients may expect to resume their previous level of activity but find that they are weak, anxious, and depressed. They may have trouble sleeping because of a fear of dying. They may feel stifled by the overprotection of their spouse, yet be afraid to be home alone.

If they perceive their health as poor, they will have a slow return to normal life. Family conflicts may occur because of changes needed in diet, activity, and medications. Some patients may not be able to return to previous jobs or to any work. Spouses and other family members may have assumed new roles in the patient's absence. Well-intentioned attempts to take over responsibilities and free the patient from pressures actually may erode the patient's self-esteem and promote family conflict (Guzzelta & Dossey, 1984).

The nurse can prepare the patient and family for this recovery period by comprehensive teaching started several days before the patient's discharge. The patient and the patient's spouse should be present so they hear the same instructions and can ask questions. A group class is helpful for patients with similar problems so that families can learn from one another.

Patients and families need to know about anticipated emotional responses and to plan how to handle these responses without hurting others. Instructions on diet, activity, and medications should be given. Spouses need to understand the instructions, but they should not nag the competent patients to follow the instructions. Follow-up medical care also needs to be discussed.

Rehabilitation is a lifelong process. It is easier for patients to stay motivated if they have family and group support. Cooking prudent heart-healthy meals for the whole family increases compliance more than making one meal for the patient and another meal for the others. Exercise as a part of the daily routine and done with one or more persons is more successful than walking alone. Formal groups for patients (Mended Hearts) and spouses are helpful for sharing concerns and for problem solving. The AHA locally can provide information about group meetings. A family physician who maintains close contact with the patient gives assurance of an interest in the patient's welfare and increases the patient's compliance.

CONCLUSION

Psychological care of cardiac patients is a vital part of their recovery from illness. The heart symbolizes life, love, and emotions. Injury to the heart cuts to the very core of life and leaves patients and families afraid of death or of radically changed lives. Comprehensive nursing care from the acute illness through recovery will help modify the psychological stress of cardiac illness and will promote recovery for patients and their families.

EXAM QUESTIONS

CHAPTER 6
Questions 52–67

52. A type A person has just been told by a physician to cut back work hours to help decrease stress-induced hypertension. How would this person most likely respond?

    a. "I've been noticing a lot of pressure at work, and I planned to cut back."

    b. "I'm busy working on a big project. I need to work more hours, not fewer."

    c. "You're probably right. I'll give my biggest account to my partner to finish."

    d. "I'll just take a little nap after lunch and that will help with my stress."

53. Which of the following coronary-prone men most likely would see a need to follow medical orders?

    a. Fred, whose boss just had a heart attack

    b. Tom, whose neighbor just had bypass surgery

    c. Rick, who has been told he is at risk for CHD but has no signs or symptoms

    d. John, who has chest pain during stressful meetings at work

54. The most common first response of a patient to the pain of a heart attack is:

    a. Panic

    b. A call to 911

    c. Denial

    d. Anger

55. Your patient says, "You don't know what you are doing! No wonder I'm not getting well faster!" What stage of grief is this patient in?

    a. Anger

    b. Denial

    c. Bargaining

    d. Depression

56. True or false: A spouse may feel anger toward the patient who experiences a MI.

    a. True

    b. False

57. True or false: Nurses have been shown in research studies to clearly identify family needs.

    a. True

    b. False

58. Which of the following is true about patients' reactions to the diagnosis of MI?

    a. Denial often occurs during the first hour.

    b. Anger is childlike response and should be punished.

    c. Atheists will not try bargaining because they do not believe in God.

    d. Most patients accept the diagnosis quickly because the physician tells them it is true.

59. Your patient had bypass surgery 3 days ago. He screams out suddenly that the goblin is trying to get him. Your assessment of the situation tells you which of the following?

    a. He may be experiencing the confusion of ICU psychosis.

    b. He is having a nightmare and needs sedation immediately.

    c. He is mentally imbalanced and needs a psychiatric consultation.

    d. He thinks it is Halloween.

60. One way to minimize ICU psychosis is to:

    a. Leave the lights on 24 hr a day

    b. Explain all procedures before doing them

    c. Make light of frightening things patients see at other bedsides

    d. Move all equipment into the patient's visual field so the patient can see it

61. Near-death experiences may occur in which of the following groups of persons?

    a. All patients who have cardiopulmonary resuscitation

    b. Religious patients only

    c. Almost all trauma victims

    d. Persons of all cultures, classes, and occupations

62. Patients who have had a near-death experience usually say which of the following?

    a. Devils appeared to remind them of their sins.

    b. The experience was frightening and made them want to come back to life.

    c. They had a feeling of peace and serenity.

    d. They decided to take extra care with their health afterward to avoid having the experience again.

63. Patients become anxious at the time of transfer from the ICU to a ward. Which of the following might help minimize their anxiety?

    a. Sympathize with them about the lack of good care on the wards.

    b. Keep them informed of their progress and the anticipated date of transfer.

    c. Do not talk about the transfer until it is happening so that you do not get their hopes up.

    d. Tell them you will keep them in the ICU as long as possible so that they will be safe.

64. Patients waking up after heart surgery usually are concerned about:

    a. Pain

    b. Where their belongings are

    c. When they will have to do the incentive spirometer

    d. How much their chest tubes are draining

65. Studies have shown that the most important need of families of critically ill patients is:

    a. To be at the patient's bedside when the patient wakes up

    b. To have hope

    c. To have a telephone in the waiting room for calling other family members with updates on the patient's condition

    d. To have access to the patient's medical record

66. Patients who are discharged from the hospital after cardiac surgery or treatment for cardiovascular disease usually feel:

    a. Relieved that their spouse is hovering about in case the patient needs something

    b. Glad to turn over their usual responsibilities to other family members

    c. Weak, anxious, and, possibly, depressed

    d. A renewed strength to get up and entertain visitors

67. Why are group teaching methods and discussions good for cardiac patients and their families?

    a. They prevent any one patient form monopolizing the conversation.

    b. Patients and their family members can share concerns with others in similar situations.

    c. Patients can learn about several different medical problems at the same time.

    d. They give a spouse permission to have control over the home care of the patient.

CHAPTER 7

INTERVENTIONS TO REDUCE RISK FACTORS

CHAPTER OBJECTIVE

After studying this chapter, the reader will be able to discuss at least one treatment approach for the following: an obese patient, a smoker, a person with high plasma cholesterol levels, a person with elevated plasma glucose levels, an inactive patient, and one with high levels of stress.

LEARNING OBJECTIVES

After studying this chapter, the reader should be able to

1. Describe several treatment approaches to hypertension.

2. Explain two methods that can be used to help patients stop smoking.

3. Describe the two diets used for lowering plasma LDL cholesterol levels, and explain the criteria for using drug therapy.

4. List the three important phases of any exercise program, and discuss why each phase contributes to the success of the program.

5. Describe several differences between an exercise prescription for a patient at risk of CHD and one for a patient who has had an MI.

INTRODUCTION

Many programs are available for patients with risk factors for cardiovascular disease. They may involve reeducating patients about their risks, providing special programs that include support group therapy and a graduated approach to changing the behavior or factors that make patients more susceptible to the development of cardiovascular disease.

This chapter describes some of the programs and approaches available for patients who need to lose weight, increase their levels of physical fitness through exercise, stop smoking, lower cholesterol levels, combat hypertension, or reduce their elevated plasma glucose levels. In addition, one section addresses some special programs available for patients who are recovering from MIs or coronary artery bypass surgery.

Once risk factors for CHD are isolated through the history, physical examination, and special tests such as exercise ECGs, a plan of action is usually formulated to help patients change behaviors that are placing them at risk of CHD. Smokers will need to know what they can do to stop smoking. Obese patients need direction and guidance to lose weight. Hypertensive patients will have many questions and concerns about diet and medication. Sedentary patients will want to know how to "get started" on an exercise program.

Nurses can play an important role as health educators and often can help answer questions that patients have about treatment options. It is helpful to know what options are available for these patients. Once the programs are under way, patients need supportive help and encouragement to continue what, it is hoped, will be permanent changes in lifestyle and attitudes.

MANAGING HYPERTENSION

After elevated blood pressure is diagnosed, a search is usually made to find the cause. As mentioned earlier, hypertension has many possible causes, including dietary factors, obesity, alcohol abuse, central nervous system disease, and use of oral contraceptives or monoamine oxidase inhibitors.

Patients with mild hypertension may respond to simple measures such as minor changes in their diets or restriction of sodium. For many obese hypertensive patients, losing weight brings blood pressure back to normal levels. Evaluating the amount of sodium in the diet and helping the patient cut back often reduce blood pressure levels.

Finally, evaluating all the drugs the patient is taking, including over-the-counter products, may reveal an unsuspected pharmacologic cause of elevated blood pressure. Products that can contribute to hypertension include nose drops, exogenous estrogens in postmenopausal women, nonsteroidal antiinflammatory drugs, and antacids that contain sodium (Grundy et al., 1987).

Drug therapy. Most patients with diastolic pressure readings of 90 mm Hg or more should be treated with antihypertensive drugs when diet and/or sodium restriction do not reduce blood pressure. Traditionally, this has been accomplished by using a "stepped-care" approach in which agents are gradually added to the treatment regimen. In all cases, the treatment approach has to be individualized and often requires a trial period to evaluate dosages and effects from each type of medication.

Lifestyle modification to achieve normal blood pressure should be attempted initially for at least 6 months in most patients with stage 1 (mild) hypertension, especially those without associated risk factors or evidence of end-organ damage. All patients should be encouraged to maintain lifestyle changes, because they may be able to reduce the dose of drug needed to manage their hypertension.

The Joint National Committee on Detection, Evaluation and Treatment of High Blood Pressure recommends low-dose hydrochlorothiazide, 12.5–25.0 mg daily, as the initial drug of choice for patients with uncomplicated hypertension ("Fifth Report," 1993).

ß-Blocker drugs are also a preferred initial agent for the treatment of hypertension because long-term studies have shown they reduce cardiovascular morbidity and mortality. ß-blockers are contraindicated in several populations of patients, including those with bronchospastic disease, congestive heart failure, and advanced heart block and should be used with caution with diabetic patients. Examples of ß-blocker drugs include atenolol, propranolol, metoprolol and timolol.

Calcium channel blockers such as verapamil, diltiazem, and nifedipine decrease arterial blood pressure by vasodilating the vascular bed. This class of antihypertensive agents should be used cautiously with patients with congestive heart failure and should not be used at all in patients with second- or third-degree heart block.

A relatively new class of drug called angiotensin-converting enzyme inhibitors (ACE inhibitors) work by blocking the conversion of angiotensin I to angiotensin II, which is a potent vasoconstrictor. Examples of this type of agent include captopril, enalapril, and lisinopril. They should not be used in patients with real artery stenosis.

An excellent reference that includes a detailed discussion of the many types of antihypertensive agents is *Cardiovascular Medications for Cardiac Nursing* by (Underhill et al., 1990).

Improving compliance. Compliance can be a problem for many patients with essential hypertension. This is especially true for those who have no signs or symptoms. When hypertension is diagnosed on a routine physical examination, patients who have no signs or symptoms may tend to dismiss the importance of the diagnosis and thus not take their medication or only take it periodically.

Communication between the health care team and patient is extremely important and can affect the success or failure of antihypertensive therapy. Nurses can improve compliance by teaching patients about the hidden nature of hypertension. As common as it is, hypertension is not well understood by many people. Because it causes few outward signs, many patients may ignore the problem. However, if they understand the progressive nature of atherosclerosis and the effects of elevated blood pressure on the heart and vascular system, they may be more likely to take their medication and to watch sodium intake and other dietary suggestions a nurse may make.

Some patients may fail to take their medications because they are afraid of side effects. This may happen when their physician describes the possible side effects of an antihypertensive while writing out the prescription. Many physicians diligently outline every possible side effect a patient might experience. As a result, the patient tends to remember the least common and most frightening side effect, such as impotence, confusion, depression, and lupus erythematosus (Kimball, 1981). Older patients may be particularly worried about lethargy and confusion.

Patients also are subject to hearsay and rumors about high blood pressure from well-meaning family members and friends. For example, some family members or friends will suggest that "just taking it easy" or relaxing will take care of the problem. Their rationale is that emotional stress is causing the high blood pressure. Some patients are afraid of diagnostic procedures that will pinpoint their hypertension. They may be particularly worried about invasive procedures such as intravenous pyelograms or renal arteriograms. The underlying fears are fears of needles and of violation of their body image (Kimball, 1981). Other patients may have heard that all antihypertensive medications are poisonous or dangerous, or that they somehow change the body and mind. Patients may deny that they have a problem and state that it really is not important, because they have so many other important things to do. Finally, another group may complain about the cost of antihypertensive medications and opt to skip them, because they "can't really tell if the drugs are working, anyway."

Two elements that have greatly improved compliance with antihypertensive programs have been good follow-up and supportive reassurance (Kimball, 1981). This approach is especially helpful when patients with hypertension respond favorably to encouragement and react positively to good reports from healthcare professionals. Helping patients understand just what high blood pressure is and its silent but deadly nature will help counteract the rumors and hearsay from well-meaning but misinformed friends, neighbors, and family members.

Nursing guidelines for treating hypertensive patients. A few general guidelines may be helpful when working with hypertensive patients (Frohlich, 1983; Loebel & Spratto, 1983):

1. Check baseline blood pressure before starting a patient on any antihypertensive agent.

2. Regularly reassess blood pressure.

3. Obtain guidelines from the physician regarding significant blood pressure levels that should be reported for each patient.

STOP-SMOKING PROGRAMS

Tobacco is the most widely used addictive substance in the world (Cohen, 1988). Smoking cigarettes is a serious health risk and a part of their lifestyle that many smokers would like to change. Smoking is a complex habit, however, and the addictive qualities are only partially understood. The pharmacologic effects of nicotine on the body certainly play a role, mood or affective state is involved, and social influences are also powerful ingredients. Smoking may be associated with a need to relax, to relieve boredom, or to reward oneself. Smoking a cigarette is also associated with a large number of experiences in a large number of smoking situations, such as the end of meals or with a cup of coffee. It is practiced so often that smokers often are unaware of the many factors that control their smoking habit (Best & Bloch, 1979).

Each smoker has a unique set of reasons for smoking, as well as a variety of attitudes, motivations, and personality characteristics that can affect the response to treatment. Studies that have attempted to target one particular personality trait in order to help smokers quit have nearly all failed (Best & Bloch, 1979). Attempts to link motivation and expectations of success have also failed (Best, 1975).

What does work? Apparently, matching the smoker to behavior modification programs on the basis of both motivation and personality traits has been successful in some cases (Best, 1971; Bornstein et al., 1977). For example, patients who seem to have little or no commitment to stop may benefit from a commitment training program (Hildebrandt & Feldman, 1975). Others, who feel they are in control of the consequences of their habit may make better use of a self-control training manual. Anxious smokers may benefit from stress management, and so forth.

The most successful long-term programs have incorporated a number of approaches, including behavior modification, aversion training, and pharmacologic products such as nicotine chewing gum and nicotine transdermal systems. Today, as never before, a person who wants to stop smoking can choose from a variety of methods offered at private clinics, at workshops, at work, at school, and via some community-wide programs as well.

The nurse can help patients who want to stop smoking by telling them about programs available in the community and by helping refer them to such programs. There will be many opportunities to reinforce a person's stated desire to stop smoking and to suggest such programs. Then, too, when the subject comes up, it does not hurt to describe some of the many physical repercussions of smoking, such as emphysema or cardiovascular disease.

Five approaches are used to help a smoker stop:

1. Group strategies
2. Educational and attitude-change strategies
3. Pharmacologic strategies, including nicotine-containing gum and transdermal patches
4. Hypnosis
5. Behavior modification

Support groups. Group meetings are a popular setting for smoking modification and have successfully helped 15–30% of participants stop smoking (Best, 1971). The discussions, moral support, and social pressure from such groups can be extremely helpful.

Educational and attitudinal changes. Changes in health behavior often require a two-step process: first, the motivation to change, and second, taking action to change. Many individual physicians and organizations, such as the American Cancer Society and the AHA, supply abundant information in the form of handouts about the hazards of smoking. The limitation to these approaches may be that although they describe what the smoker should do, they do not tell the smoker how to quit (Best, 1971). In one study of Massachusetts physicians (Okene et al., 1988), nearly all the doctors reported that they had information on the smoking status of all new patients and had told their patients to quit. However, a much smaller number reported counseling their patients on how to stop smoking. From 3% to 16% of physicians said they were prepared to counsel smokers but reported that they needed information about where to refer patients and about the techniques that would be used at those centers. They also reported they could use much more training in counseling and referring smokers.

Despite certain limitations, however, the widespread use of antismoking campaigns seem to be working. The prevalence of smoking has declined in the last 30 years from 40% to 29% of the population (Pierce et al., 1989). These campaigns have certainly made it far more difficult for smokers to smoke with ease in restaurants, hospitals, movie theaters, and airplanes. This undoubtedly has helped some smokers quit.

Pharmacologic approaches. With the exception of nicotine gum and transdermal systems (patches), most pharmacologic approaches to stopping smoking have not worked well. The first product marketed, lobeline sulfate, available as Bantron or Nikoban, is offered as a way to help smokers abstain during initial withdrawal from cigarettes. However, the effects of such products are both weak and temporary and often are no more helpful than placebos. Efforts to use smokeless tobacco have generally been met with the criticism that a dependency similar to that in cigarette smokers develops in those who use it (Benowitz, 1988). In addition, the health hazards known to be caused by cigarette smoking and suspected to be related to long-term exposure to nicotine are expected to pose a hazard in those who use smokeless tobacco as well.

Hypnosis. Since 1980, the American Psychiatric Association has recognized nicotine dependence and nicotine withdrawal as diagnostic entities. Hypnosis is one of the psychiatric techniques used to help smokers quit (Cohen, 1988). Hypnosis may seem to be a drastic approach to stopping smoking, but its success rates have varied from 60% to 100% (Watkins, 1976). Hypnosis may also be used to teach alternative behaviors to use in situations in which a cigarette might be desired, for example, in dealing with tension, anger, or a desire to have something to do with the hands.

Behavior modification. Because smoking is often characterized as a chain of behaviors and events, modifying this chain through a number of steps has been successful for many patients. One of the most common techniques is aversion therapy. This approach works on the principle that situations lead to smoking because they have become associated with smoking through experience and because smoking in such settings has been rewarding to the smoker. Aversive conditioning attempts to create an urge not to smoke in these situations. Some have used electric shock. For the most part, this has not been effective, except when self-management techniques are combined with the shock.

A number of other approaches, all of which are practiced only under careful medical supervision, have been tried. Rapid smoking, or aversive oversmoking, is another approach that has been used to try to help smokers break the habit. This method entails having a smoker sit down, at first once a day and then gradually less often, and chain-smoke as many cigarettes as possible, taking puffs every 6sec (Lichtenstein et al., 1973). Clients are instructed to abstain from smoking between sessions. With a good relationship between the instructor and smoker/ex-smoker, success rates of up to 100% at termination of the program and 60% up to 6 months later have been reported. Rapid smoking apparently works best when done in a laboratory setting, rather than at home, and also when treatment is continued until the client is abstinent and reporting little or no difficulty controlling the urge to smoke.

Covert sensitization is another aversive technique. In this technique, smokers are asked repeatedly to imagine themselves in a typical smoking situation and to conjure up vivid, powerful negative consequences, for example, becoming nauseated at the sight of a cigarette and throwing up on the package (Cautela, 1970). This approach has apparently worked best in combination with rapid smoking (Severson & Hynd, 1977).

Stimulus control is another approach that attempts to interrupt the usual cues that stimulate a smoker to pick up a cigarette. Two steps are usually involved: restricting smoking to a few, often unusual, cues to stop associations with previous smoking situations and gradually reducing smoking, even in the presence of the cues. All sorts of devices have been used, including locking cigarette boxes that could be opened only at designated times and pocket timers. Other techniques involve planned nonsmoking intervals or specific times or even specific settings when smoking is allowed. Results have been mixed, but generally not too successful.

Another type of behavior modification involves using consequence techniques. These techniques seek to intercept the urge to smoke at the point in the smoking chain when a smoker decides to smoke. A therapist might suggest several nonsmoking techniques a patient could substitute for smoking. For example, if a person has a strong urge to smoke while at a party, he or she would be urged to substitute an action for the cigarette. In this case, this might entail going for a short walk until the urge passed (Best, 1971). Or, contingency management might be tried. This is a process of assessing a monetary penalty for smoking or giving some sort of reward for not smoking. This

approach has produced fairly successful short-term results.

Many have found that a combination of these techniques provides the greatest success. Recently, some communities have set up programs for residents who wish to stop smoking. In one community, a program based on education, behavior modification, and group support led to a permanent smoking cessation rate of 22% after 1 year (Hurt et al., 1988). Factors that seemed to lead to success included having a white-collar occupation, having stopped before for more than 1 month, being male, and wanting to stop smoking because of health concerns.

The Stanford Stop Smoking Project used a trial of nicotine polacrilex and self-administered relapse prevention materials in a group of 600 volunteers (Fortmann et al., 1988), stressing a "minimal contact" approach. Eight self-help relapse prevention modules were mailed weekly. Then, nicotine-containing gum was used either freely whenever the urge to smoke occurred or on a fixed, hourly schedule, where 12 pieces per day were consumed. After 6 months, 31% of volunteers who used the gum and received the modules had abstained from smoking.

A number of companies have also started anti-smoking programs for their employees. One example is Johnson & Johnson's Live for Life program, part of the company's overall wellness program (Shipley et al., 1988). At branches of the company that offered the Live for Life program, 22.6% of smokers quit. The quit rate was particularly high among employees who were at high risk for CHD. Thirty-two percent of all high-risk smokers quit smoking after participating in the program. This study showed that company-wide smoking cessation efforts can be effective.

Thus, most successful programs use a combination of approaches, after tailoring the approach to the individual patient. What works for one patient will not automatically work for another.

LOWERING CHOLESTEROL LEVELS

When a patient has high LDL cholesterol levels, the immediate treatment goal is to reduce cholesterol levels. The desired level depends on the presence of other risk factors. For example, in persons with no CHD risk factors, LDL cholesterol should be reduced to less than 160 mg/dL. For those who have at least one definite CHD risk factor, the goal should be to reduce LDL cholesterol levels to less than 130 mg/dL.

The current plasma cholesterol level should also be used to determine the choice of therapy. Patients who meet the criteria for active medical therapy should first undergo diet therapy to reduce LDL cholesterol levels. The goal of diet therapy is to reduce elevated blood cholesterol levels while still maintaining good nutrition.

Before any treatment program is undertaken, the results from cholesterol testing must be evaluated. Once the results are verified, possible secondary causes ruled out, and the patient's overall risk factor profile established (how many other risk factors for CHD are present), the initial diet can be designed.

AMERICAN HEART ASSOCIATION RECOMMENDATIONS

Step-One diet. The first step of diet therapy calls for reducing the intake of total dietary fat to 30% or less of total daily calories. Next, saturated fats should be reduced so that they make up less than 10% of total calories, and cholesterol should be reduced to less than 300 mg/day (AHA, 1990).

This Step-One Diet can be maintained for 3 months with recommended cholesterol checks at 6 weeks and 3 months. If the goals have not been reached, then a more restricted diet, Step-Two, may

be recommended.

Step-Two diet. The Step-Two diet is similar to the first one, except that saturated fats are reduced even further, to less than 7% of daily calories, and dietary cholesterol is reduced to less than 200 mg/day. Total fat intake can remain at 30% of calories, and the balance is supplied by polyunsaturated and monounsaturated fats.

When the patient is on the Step-Two diet, total cholesterol levels are measured again, and the ability to stay on the diet is reassessed at 6 weeks and then at 3 months of therapy. If patients have reached their goals, long-term monitoring can begin. If not, drug therapy may be recommended. For most patients, a trial period of 6 months of diet and counseling is attempted before drug therapy is used.

Saturated fats. Lowering saturated fat may be the most important element in the LDL cholesterol-lowering diet. The most important source of saturated fat in the diet of adult Americans is red meat: beef, pork, and lamb. The second most important is dairy fat: cheese, butter, whole milk, and ice cream. Other sources of saturated fats, such as coconut oil and cashew nuts, are not as important.

Lowering cholesterol. Cholesterol is found only in animal products. Egg yolk, which provides about 250 mg of cholesterol per yolk is the largest single source of cholesterol for Americans. Other foods that are high in cholesterol include red meats, poultry, milk, butter, and cheese. A diet that lowers cholesterol can also have measurable, positive effects on weight, VLDL levels, plasma glucose, and HDL levels. Most LDL cholesterol-lowering diets involve slight increases in the ratio of polyunsaturated fats to saturated fats. Increasing the intake of polyunsaturated fat lowers serum cholesterol. *(See Appendix.)*

Drug therapy. When diet does not alter LDL cholesterol levels, drug therapy is considered. Patients who are good candidates include those with LDL cholesterol levels of 190 mg/dL or higher without any other risk factors for CHD and those who have LDL cholesterol levels of 160 mg/dL and two other risk factors, such as overweight and hypertension.

The drugs of first choice for treating elevated LDL cholesterol levels are bile acid sequestrants, such as cholestyramine resin (Questran, Quemid) and colestipol resin (Colestid) (AHA, 1987). Nicotinic acid is preferable for patients who have triglyceride levels higher than 250 mg/dL, because bile acid sequestrants tend to raise triglyceride levels.

Cholestyramine or colestipol commonly cause gastrointestinal side effects, such as constipation, gastrointestinal upset, and malabsorption of fat-soluble vitamins such as A, D, and K. Using stool softeners or increasing fluid intake will counteract this. Other strategies are to take other drugs at least 30 min before or 4 hr after cholestyramine, always in liquid or pulpy fruit, never dry. The major side effects to watch for are fecal impaction and bleeding due to vitamin K deficiency. Nicotinic acid commonly causes flushing, headache, postural hypotension, elevated uric acid, and skin disorders, and its major side effects include glucose intolerance, liver dysfunction, and activation of peptic ulcer.

A new class of drugs for lowering LDL cholesterol are the HMG CoA reductase inhibitors. They are effective and cause fewer short-term side effects than the first group mentioned. Their long-term effects are still being studied, and thus they should be used with caution. Other drugs include probucol (Lorelco) and clofibrate (Atromid-S).

Once the maximal response to drug therapy has been achieved, patients should have initial follow-up visits at least once every 4 months, to check their responses and to note any side effects. Lipoprotein analysis should be done once a year, and total cholesterol levels should be measured at other visits. Patients on drug therapy commonly have at least a 15% reduction in LDL cholesterol (AHA, 1987). Low-fat diets must be continued when the patient is taking these medications.

Patient education. Lifestyle changes do not happen overnight. Patients who understand the importance of lowering serum lipid levels have a much better chance of sticking to a diet aimed at reducing and controlling such levels.

To meet the daily dietary goal of obtaining 10% of calories from saturated fat, and thus to reduce LDL cholesterol levels, a patient who consumes 2,500 calories each day must watch the amounts of beef, pork, lamb, or cheese consumed. Ideally, servings of these items should be kept to about 3 oz not more than five times a week, or a total of 15 oz per week. For the stricter limits of 5% saturated fat daily, no more than two or three servings of 3–4 oz of meat or cheese should be consumed per week.

One way to make this easier is to give the patient a simple quota for the number and serving size of meat or cheese meals each week. Remember that the savings in saturated fat the patient achieves by eating less red meat can be nullified by eating large amounts of dairy products high in butter fat. For example, a double dip of rich ice cream (8 oz) has just as much saturated fat (13 g) as a 3-oz steak or a 4-oz pork chop. Two tablespoons of butter provide as much fat as 24 oz of whole milk or 2 oz of baking chocolate (Podell & Stewart, 1983).

A food diary kept by patients, in which they record what they eat, the times they eat, and the amounts they eat can be helpful for determining how much fat patients are actually consuming. If they cannot or will not keep a diary, the nurse can roughly estimate intake of saturated fat by asking a few questions, such as the following:

1. How often do you eat meat or cheese? What is the typical portion size?

2. How many times a week do you think you eat ice cream, cake, or other sweets?

3. Do you drink milk every day? Is it whole milk, 2%, or skim milk?

4. How many times a week do you eat poultry, fish, or vegetables as the main course for a meal?

Nurses can play an important role in helping patients understand that high cholesterol and triglyceride levels are linked to a high risk of heart disease and that making changes in the diet helps reduce the risk of serious heart disease. Patients also need to have good follow-up so that health care professionals can intercept problems or answer questions.

LOWERING PLASMA GLUCOSE LEVELS

Cardiovascular disease is the No. 1 cause of death in diabetic patients; therefore, preventive management of diabetes is critical (Podell, 1983). Not only does diabetes itself place a person at greater risk of CHD, but the risk is also increased by coexisting risk factors. Once the diagnosis of diabetes is made, elevated plasma glucose levels (140 mg/dL) on two occasions after an overnight fast, most patients are candidates for either diet or drug therapy.

Management of diabetes is aimed at controlling hyperglycemia by diet, nutritional management, oral hypoglycemic agents, or insulin injections. Often dietary changes alone reduce plasma glucose levels. For some patients, tighter control of glucose levels with drugs is required. Using insulin enables the patient to avoid ketoacidosis and other signs and symptoms resulting from hyperglycemia.

Self-monitoring methods have enabled patients to measure plasma glucose at home. These include Chemstrip blood glucose visual quantitation and Dextrostix measurements with a reflectance meter.

Recent studies have shown the benefits of changes in lifestyle, such as weight reduction and increased exercise, to help reduce the risk of CHD in diabetic patients. Some have also suggested that health care professionals focus attention on the personality traits of patients with diabetes and try, when possible, to understand the psychological impact of the disease on the patient. This will have an effect on compliance and on the course of treatment. Patients who are told they are diabetic go through a number of stages, beginning with shock at the diagnosis and then denial, which may be manifested as a refusal to accept treatment or to follow a diet. The health care team often has to adopt a quiet watchfulness until the patient reaches acceptance of the disease; then treatment can proceed.

Chase Patterson Kimball, professor of psychiatry and medicine at the University of Chicago (1981), suggests a number of steps that may be helpful when working with a diabetic patient:

1. Remember that the individual and the disease are not separate entities, but are intimately related. The earlier the onset of the disease, the more interrelated the disease and the developing personality are. Therefore, nurses and physicians are treating the patient, not just the disease.

2. Both onset and exacerbation of diabetes are often related to psychosocial events. Managing the disease well often depends on paying attention to these other factors.

3. The effect of diabetes on the patient's life depends on many factors, including age at onset, severity of disease, personality, and professional and social responsibilities.

4. When the patient can not adapt to the diagnosis, specific psychiatric illnesses may develop that require treatment in their own right. The most common pattern is depression.

5. Remember to watch for transient or long-term

deficits in perception and cognition.

DIETS:
A WORLD OF CHOICES

The obese patient has a cornucopia of weight- loss choices, ranging from support groups that hold weekly meetings and weigh-ins to private diet clinics, hospital-based fasting programs, and gastric surgical techniques for extreme cases. Every library contains dozens of diet books outlining yet another diet approach that is a "sure" way to lose weight. Unfortunately, most of these "miracle cures" do not work because they do not give patients a way to **keep weight off** once it is lost (if it is lost). As with other treatment plans, a diet prescription must be tailored to the individual patient and his or her lifestyle, with an emphasis on permanently changing eating and exercise patterns that have resulted in obesity.

Most obese people who are at risk for cardiovascular disease have several problems in addition to obesity that require lifestyle changes to lower their risk. The best approach is multifaceted, including a low-calorie diet, moderate exercise, behavior modification, and stress management.

A diet for a healthier lifestyle. Often nurses can design a healthy diet specifically for an individual patient. Any dietary plan should be individualized, because each patient has special nutritional needs. Some need to lose weight, whereas others need to change their current diets to gain missing nutrients. Elderly patients have special needs because physiologic changes in organ systems, problems with chewing foods because of loss of teeth or poorly fitting dentures, loss of appetite, and the effects of social isolation work against a well-balanced diet. Organizations such as the AHA, which has local branches in nearly every major city, can provide helpful and healthful dietary guidelines.

Most reducing diets attempt to decrease calories to a level that is low enough to produce a steady, gradual weight loss. Generally, a good reducing diet allows a person to cut about 1,000 calories from the usual daily intake. For most patients whose weight is in the moderate range and who are fairly active, a 1,200-calorie diet for women and a 1,800-calorie diet for men leads to a loss of about a pound a week. A more restrictive diet, such as 800–1,000 calories each day, works for patients who are sedentary. By eliminating soft drinks, alcohol, fatty and sugary desserts, snack foods, table fats, and sugar, many people eliminate 500 calories from the daily diet.

The physician or nurse should prescribe a diet that provides a balance of protein, fat, and carbohydrates. Most Americans have diets that supply about two fifths of total calories from carbohydrate and fat and somewhat less than one fifth from protein (Podell, 1983). Sometimes diets high in protein and low in fat or carbohydrates are used for treating simple obesity on a crash basis. However, they are not suitable for a patient who needs long-term diet modification.

A good dietary plan provides adequate amounts of protein, fats, and carbohydrates. *(see Appendix).* The diet should also be designed so that the patient has an adequate supply of food evenly during the day to take care of energy needs. When patients report that certain times of the day are a problem for them—such as late nights, when they binge on foods—low-calorie snacks can be planned. Remember also that the need for energy declines progressively throughout adult life (Frankle & Yang, 1988).

Proteins are the major structural components of animals cells. Proteins in the diet provide the essential amino acids to replace enzymes and structural proteins in tissue (AHA, 1986). Protein is the only substance that is capable of building and repairing cells and tissues and is the major component of muscles, blood, brain, skin, nails, and internal organs, including the brain and the heart. Allowing 0.6 mg/kg per day of high-quality protein covers the needs of most healthy people. Another way to estimate this is to allow 1 g of protein per day for each 2 lb of body weight. Protein intake above 2 g/kg of body weight is not warranted. When the essential requirements are met, eating large quantities of meat does not help build large muscle. The excess ends up as an undesirably large supply of saturated fats (AHA, 1986).

Currently, Americans are consuming about 15–20% of their calories as saturated fats. As noted earlier, intake of saturated fat has been correlated with serum cholesterol values and CHD in many epidemiologic studies (AHA, 1986). Dietary fat serves as a carrier for fat-soluble vitamins and also provides essential fatty acids. There is no specific requirement for fat in the diet, and nutritional needs can be met by a diet containing 15–25 g of appropriate fats. A reducing diet should contain less than 30% of calories as fats. This amount is further broken down by types of fats. Ideally, the mix should be10% saturated fats, 10% monounsaturated fats, and 10% polyunsaturated fats. Dieters are usually warned to avoid fats because foods such as butter, margarine, and cooking oils are so high in calories that even overlooking a small step in cooking, such as incorrectly measuring margarine, can add 100–150 calories to the diet (Simonson & Heilman, 1983).

Carbohydrates provide the body's main fuel source. Carbohydrates also help in numerous body functions, digestion, and muscle exertion. Carbohydrates provide the energy needed for body work and, in most cultures, supply most of the daily energy requirements. A minimum of 150 g of digestible carbohydrate should be provided in the diet daily. Foods such as whole-grain cereals, fruits, and vegetables are prime sources of carbohydrates. A good reducing diet should contain 50 g of carbohydrate, or 1 g for every 3 lb of ideal body weight, whichever is higher. In addition, about half of the day's calories should be derived from carbohydrates.

Natural foods high in complex carbohydrates are usually low in caloric density and contain a variety of vitamins and minerals as well (AHA, 1986). In addition, more soluble and insoluble but indigestible carbohydrates, or fiber, are present in such foods. Fiber, including cellulose, lignin, gums, and pectins, is another important component of any diet plan. For the general population, fiber found in wheat, bran, and other grains is recommended (Frankle & Yang, 1988). There is growing evidence that certain soluble fibers, such as pectin, guar, and oat bran, help lower serum cholesterol levels (AHA, 1986). Moderately increasing the dietary fiber by adding oats, barley, and dried beans to the diet have been helpful for patients with high blood cholesterol levels. Too-high levels of fiber can interfere with the absorption of minerals. A safe level to aim for is 20–30 g/day.

Most dietary plans call for a daily multivitamin capsule. As a brief review, the recommended daily allowances for vitamins are as follows:

Calcium	800 mg (some have recommended higher doses for women)
Iron	12 mg
Vitamin A	5,000 IU
Vitamin D	400 IU
Thiamine	1.0 mg
Riboflavin	1.5 mg
Niacin	10.0 mg
Vitamin C	75.0 mg

Many have found that having an exchange system, or a method that allows choosing different types of foods within the same category, provides flexibility in the diet and avoids boredom. Table 11 shows types of food exchanges and portions allowed for each in a sample diet plan.

Finally, do not forget to add a prescription for water. Drinking plenty of water is one of the easiest and least expensive things a patient can do to improve overall health. On most diet plans, dieters are instructed to drink at least eight 8-oz glasses of water each day; drinking more than 10 glasses a day may flush out vitamins and minerals, leading to electrolyte imbalance. Patients with a history of renal insuffiency or congestive heart failure should obtain fluid guidelines from their physicians.

Referring the patient. Some physicians prefer to refer patients to a dietitian who can design an individual diet that supplies the necessary daily nutrients and requirements for a reducing diet and that also reduces other risk factors. The dietitian can then follow up the patient and keep the physician up to date on the patient's progress. A qualified dietitian can be found by contacting the American Dietetic Association, 430 North Michigan Avenue, Chicago, IL 60611, or by checking the local Yellow Pages.

Support groups. Groups such as Weight Watchers, Take Pounds Off Sensibly (T.O.P.S.), or Overeaters Anonymous offer diet plans plus the support of other dieters. Generally, meetings are held weekly, and members pay a fee to join. At Weight Watchers, members are weighed once a week and follow a balanced diet and exercise program and then enter a "maintenance" program designed to help them keep the pounds off.

Overeaters Anonymous is patterned after Alcoholics Anonymous. Members are urged to share their frustrations and successes at regular meetings while they lose weight on a very-restricted-calorie diet.

Diet clinics. A number of very successful diet clinics have sprung up around the country. Many offer a very-low-calorie diet (500 calories/day), plus daily weigh-ins and counseling. After the client has lost weight, he or she follows a program of gradually adding calories back to reach a stabi-lized diet.

Hospital fasts. For extremely obese persons, a supervised liquid fasting program, such as the Optifast program, may be the answer. With this program, patients consume measured amounts of liquid protein until an ideal weight is reached. Patients are closely supervised and have ready counseling during difficult periods. Because of the limited calories, patients lose large amounts of weight quickly. The restrictions of the diet also lead to a high dropout rate.

University-based programs. Nearly every large medical center offers a weight-loss program. A few of the better known programs are those at Duke University, Johns Hopkins University, and Vanderbilt University. Duke University is the home of the Rice Diet developed more than 45 years ago by Walter Kempner. Meals consist of fresh fruit, cooked rice, and noncaloric beverages. Patients lose up to 12 lb the first week, and often 5–7 lb each week afterward, until they reach a weight that is often lower than that suggested by life insurance charts. The drawback to this diet is that it is bland and boring. Also, once a patient leaves the controlled setting, he or she may regain the lost pounds (Moscovitz, 1986).

The University Medical Diet, designed at Johns Hopkins University, uses reeducation about foods and the role of exercise to help patients lose weight and keep it off for good. After patients undergo a series of tests to evaluate the factors that have led to obesity, they are given an individualized diet that basically provides 20% protein, 30% fat, and 50% carbohydrate. This program also stresses adding an exercise program to help speed up weight loss and to keep weight off once it is lost (Simonson & Heilman, 1983).

Behavior modification. Regardless of what program a patient enters, that person must modify his or her eating behavior if the weight is to stay off. Many factors influence eating behavior, including biologic, psychological, sociocultural, and environmental cues.

One of the simpler yet effective methods for helping patients understand what they eat, when they eat, and the situations that make them hungry is to have them keep a food diary for at least 3 days, and ideally for 1–2 weeks. Patients record what is eaten, the time and setting, and the mood that accompanied eating. The dietitian or therapist can then analyze the diary to see the factors that may be causing overeating. (Many support groups, including Weight Watchers and diet clinics, also use food diaries.)

Table 11

Food Exchanges

For Women *(1,200 calories)*	**For Men** *(1,500 calories)*
Fruit (3)	Fruit (4– 6)
Vegetables (2 at least)	Vegetables (2 at least)
Milk (2)	Milk (2)
Bread (2–3)	Bread (4– 5)
Fat (3)	Fat (3)
Protein (6– 8)	Protein (8–10)

Optional: up to 550 calories/week for men and women

Note: This food plan provides about 50% of calories from carbohydrate, 20% from protein, and 30% from fat; it also provides 155 g of carbohydrate, 65 g of protein, 45 g of fat, 300 mg of cholesterol, and 2,000 mg of sodium.

AN EXERCISE PRESCRIPTION

Despite a nationwide emphasis on fitness, the average American is still far less fit than he or she should be, largely as a result of our sedentary lifestyle. Years of lack of fitness lead to a host of chronic health problems. The benefits of regular vigorous exercise are well documented. The study of Harvard alumni mentioned earlier is a good example (Paffenberger et al., 1978). In that study, persons who exercised only once in a while had a 64% greater risk of heart disease than fellow alumni who exercised vigorously and often or who expended more than 2,000 calories/week in vigorous exercise.

Regular vigorous exercise also has a powerful effect on the blood vessels and blood chemistry. Regular exercise helps increase blood oxygen content, increases blood cell mass and blood volume, increases the efficiency of peripheral blood distribution and return, increases blood supply to muscles, and leads to a more efficient exchange of oxygen and carbon dioxide levels. It also helps reduce serum triglyceride levels and LDL cholesterol levels, decreases systolic and diastolic blood pressure, and reduces glucose intolerance (Cantu, 1980). Maximal oxygen uptake, or aerobic capacity, is an important measure of physical fitness. As discussed in chapter 6, special equipment can be used during treadmill stress testing or bicycle ergometry to analyze the oxygen and carbon dioxide content of expired air and to determine maximal and submaximal oxygen uptake (Getchell, 1979). Maximal uptake is used to measure fitness in young patients, whereas submaximal testing is safer for older or sedentary adults.

Exercise also contributes to a general overall sense of well-being, helps reduce anxiety, and improves body image. It can help reduce a tendency to depression, and for many serious runners can produce a sense of exhilaration and energy.

A well-designed exercise plan can increase a patient's aerobic capacity by 20% to 30%, can improve cardiac and respiratory function, enhance muscle strength, and improve flexibility (Chung, 1986). Once-sedentary patients are often surprised at the fitness levels they can achieve after a relatively short period of gradually increasing exercise.

In contrast, improperly designed exercise programs or too-vigorous sports may be harmful to some people (Chung, 1986). Any exercise program or sport that requires a workload beyond the person's current physical capacity, determined by the exercise ECG, is harmful and can even be life threatening for cardiac patients whose physical capacity is severely limited. For example, jogging on a very cold or very hot day can be hazardous for any person, not only a person who has CHD (Chung, 1986).

Although most nurses are familiar with the importance of exercise, as in the case of range of motion for bedridden patients or the benefits of early ambulation for the postcardiac patient, the concept of promoting physical fitness for protecting health and preventing disease is still largely ignored in nursing schools curriculum (Pender, 1987). As a result, many nurses are uncomfortable with designing an exercise program for patients.

All nurses should be able to evaluate a patient's physical fitness level and to apply their knowledge of physiology, chemistry, and anatomy, as well as cardiovascular data, to help the patient get started and stay on an exercise program. Many nurses are designing and providing weight-control and exercise programs for adults in the community and for children through school-based programs.

DETERMINING EXERCISE CAPACITY

The results of physical examination, family history, blood lipid profile, resting blood pressure, resting ECGs, and exercise ECGs, are used to estimate the patient's risk and general overall physical fitness. In addition, target heart rates can be used to establish a baseline, and to chart the patient's progress. Remember, too, many people overestimate the amount of exercise they get each day, and if they kept an exercise diary akin to a foods diary, they would be surprised at how little vigorous exercise they get each day. Remember to advise your patients to obtain permission from their physicians to start an exercise program.

A good exercise program should have the fol-

lowing characteristics (Cantu, 1980):

1. The exercise should be enjoyable.

2. The exercise should be vigorous enough so that the patient expends at least 400 calories per session (except for patients who have had an MI).

3. The exercise should keep the heart rate at 70–85% of the patient's maximum potential for 20–30 min (or about 120–150 beats per minute).

4. The exercise should be rhythmical, allowing the muscles to alternately contract and relax.

5. The exercise should be repeated for 30–60 min, three to five times a week.

6. The exercise should be systematically integrated into the patient's lifestyle.

Some of the exercises that can be used to achieve the target heart rate and thus develop cardiopulmonary and muscular endurance include running, swimming, cross-country skiing, cycling, rowing, handball, and squash. For many persons, brisk walking is an activity that they can easily adapt, wherever they may live and whatever their occupation is. In fact, walking is universally recognized as one of the best exercises available to people of all ages.

Each stage in the exercise prescription should be carefully explained, including the time, frequency of repetition, and any warning signs or symptoms that call for stopping the exercise. Just as with most medications, it is easy for patients to forget the "exercise prescription," after a few days, and it may be helpful to write down the types and extent of exercise, explaining them as clearly as possible. Other patients, particularly type A persons or those who are time or achievement oriented, may try to do too much, too fast, and too soon and may be impatient with the fact that all successful exercise programs involve slow and steady progress. As Pender noted (1987), such people assume that if walking at 5 km/hr is good for the heart, a run at 15 km is three times better, and a time-saver as well! Just as with individual diet approaches, certain exercise approaches work better for some patients than for others. Some gregarious patients might do better in a twice-weekly aerobics class where classmates and instructor can be supportive and helpful. Other people might enjoy the solitude of exercising alone or with family members only. However, there is one thing to remember: Older and coronary-prone people should not exercise alone, if possible, for obvious reasons.

The type of activity should be available near home or office, and when it is possible, exercise should be built into the daily routine. A secretary can walk briskly to the subway or bus in the morning and use the stairs rather than the elevator. In the evenings, patients might be encouraged to ride their bicycles to the store or to walk. Before any sport or exercise program is undertaken, patients should be taught to monitor their heart rates.

The heart-rate method. The heart-rate method of monitoring exercise is based on the relationship between the person's heart rate and the amount of oxygen consumed. When a patient is exercising at a rate that provides maximal intake of oxygen, the maximally obtainable heart rate is also achieved. A physically fit person usually has a lower heart rate and more rapid recovery, or return to resting heart rate, than a person who is not physically fit.

Table 12

Target Heart Rates For Different Ages

Age (yr)	Target Heart Rates / Maximum Oxygen Uptake (%)			
20–30	118 (80)	145 (74)	164 (84)	195 (100)
30–40	118 (63)	141 (75)	158 (86)	188 (100)
40–50	116 (65)	137 (77)	153 (86)	178 (100)
50–60	114 (67)	133 (78)	145 (85)	171 (100)
60–70	111 (68)	129 (79)	141 (87)	163 (100)

Source: Shephard, R. J. (1983). Exercise and primary prevention of coronary heart disease. In R. N. Podell & M. M. Stewart (Eds.), *Primary Prevention of Coronary Heart Disease* (p. 219). Menlo Park, CA: Addison-Wesley.

Maximal heart rate can be measured directly during a maximal stress test, or it can be predicted from data obtained from charts based on studies of many healthy men and women. The maximal heart rate is usually predicted by using the following formula: 220 minus age in years. The problem with this formula is that is seriously underestimates the maximal rate for healthy older North Americans (Shephard, 1983). Many use a simple table, such as *Table 12*, to estimate an individual's target heart rate. This table is only a general guide, because values vary greatly from person to person and are marginally higher in young women than in young men. Maximal heart rate may also be impossible to measure because the onset of symptoms or signs may stop testing. Finally, maximal heart rates may be depressed by drugs, such as ß-blockers, or by exposure to high altitudes (Shephard, 1983).

Target heart rate is usually introduced in terms of lower and upper limits. The lower limit is the least intensity of effort required to produce endurance training. The upper limit is designed to act as a safety net to help patients avoid a cardiac problem. The target heart rate can actually be expressed as a percentage of the maximal rate. That is, a middle-aged man might be advised to exercise to at least 60% of his maximal oxygen uptake, but not more than 75%.

Patients should first master the technique of getting a reasonably accurate pulse count (70–75 beats per minute for the average person) while resting. They can do this for a 30-sec period. The count must be timed accurately. In the beginning, patients should check their pulse and then have a trained health care worker take it to see that they know how to take it correctly.

FIVE IMPORTANT PARTS OF ANY EXERCISE PROGRAM

Once patients know how to take their pulse rate, the five parts of the exercise prescription can be taught: proper breathing, stretching and limbering-up exercises, a warm-up period, the endurance exercise period, and a cooling-down period.

Breathing. Breathing is such a natural process. Why should a person be concerned about breathing? Proper breathing techniques can greatly enhance any exercise program and help supply adequate oxygen to the muscles, brain, and other parts of the body. Proper breathing is not just a matter of inhaling or exhaling; it includes expanding the lungs and using proper posture to make lung expansion possible (Pender, 1987). Because of space limitations, this text does not review the physiology of breathing, but it does give a few breathing exercises you can teach to patients before they embark on their new exercise program.

Two exercises you might try with patients are the Nikolaus breathing technique (Isaacs & Kobles, 1978) and diaphragmatic breathing (Everly & Girdano, 1980). The Nickolaus technique helps a patient become more aware of breathing patterns and gain control of breathing, increases lung capacity, and also relaxes the entire body in preparation for exercise. Here is the technique: The patient lies on the floor on a rug or mat, with knees bent, keeping the lower back pressed against the floor. The feet are 6 to 8 in. apart. Toes are turned slightly in so that the arches are lifted. The chin is kept toward the chest, and the mouth is slightly open. Patients are advised to imagine that they are lying in bed, about to fall asleep, relaxed, with all cares and worries "released." The hands are placed on the stomach with the middle fingers meeting at the navel so

the patient can feel the up and downward movement of the abdominal muscles. The patient then breathes slowly through the nose, counting to four, letting the diaphragm fall and the abdomen rise. The breath should flow upward into the chest, expanding the upper part of the torso. Then the air should be released through the nose and mouth, gently contracting the muscles of the chest, then the abdomen. As the abdomen contracts, the lower back should make contact with the floor. The exercise should be repeated six times.

Diaphragmatic breathing can be done while sitting in a straight-back chair. First, the patient assumes a comfortable position, with the feet resting flat on the floor and hands placed one over the other at the navel. The eyes should remain open. Then patients imagine a giant balloon in the abdomen beneath their hands that they are trying to fill with air. The hands will rise as the imaginary balloon is filled. The patient should continue inhaling through the nose until the imaginary balloon is filled to the top. The total time for inhalation should be about 5–7 sec. It's a good idea to inhale through the nose because this allows the air to be warmed and moistened and for impurities to be removed. Also, air inhaled through the mouth may be too cold for deep breathing. The air should be held while the phrase "I feel calm" is repeated slowly; then the air can be exhaled to empty the balloon. During exhalation, the raised abdomen and chest recede. Patients can use this breathing exercise four to five times at a setting at least 8 or 10 times a day. If the patient complains about feeling light-headed, the number of cycles can be reduced.

Stretching exercises. Stretching exercises enable the patient to improve flexibility and help avoid muscle and tendon injury. In some overly vigorous programs for sedentary middle-aged adults, as many as 50% of recruits have been disabled by musculoskeletal injuries or problems (Shephard, 1983).

All stretches should be held for 10–15 sec for maximum benefit and should be held at the point of mild discomfort, not pain. Some of the stretching exercises a patient can use include the following:

- Arm circles: 10 outward, 10 inward, 10 forward, 10 backward

- Touching the opposite toe (10 on each side)

- Side stretches (5 on each side)

- Leg-overs (5 on each side)

- Low back stretching: while lying down, lift knee to chest (5 times on each side)

- Hamstring stretches (3 times on each side). Patient sits down, grasps an ankle with both hands, and then leans over until the head touches the corresponding knee.

- Achilles tendon stretches (3 times on each side). Patient stands 3 f in front of a wall, leans forward, and places the palms on the wall.

These are but a few exercises. Many others can be found in a number of textbooks, including an excellent exercise prescription book by B. Getchell, *Physical Fitness: A Way of Life* (John Wiley & Sons, 1979).

Warm-up exercises. A warm-up period allows the patient to begin exercising at a comfortable rate, to warm the muscles, and to gradually increase oxygen intake. It raises the temperature in active muscles by 2°–4°F, produces active local vasodilation, and reduces the viscosity of muscle fibers. The warm-up period usually lasts 5–10 min, until the desired intensity of exercise is reached. An example of a warming-up exercise might be walking moderately and progressing through fast walking to the intended jogging speed. Other types of warm-up exercises might be walking briskly for 30 sec, jogging for 45 sec, doing arm circles, doing jumping jacks, or doing floor or wall push-ups.

Endurance exercise. Endurance exercise is defined as vigorous but not excessively strenuous activity that involves the large muscles of the body. It is the most important part of an exercise prescription. Endurance exercise lessens the workload on the heart by subsequent vigorous exercise. It also helps burn excess body fat. After 3–5 min of endurance exercise, patients should check their pulse and adjust the exercise rate if the pulse is not in the target zone. Endurance exercise lasts 30 min per session, although some people may need to work up to this amount of time over several weeks. The minimum intensity for a training effect is about 60% of maximum oxygen intake, or less if the patient has been bedfast for some weeks. The maximum goal for a sedentary person is about 70–75% of maximum oxygen intake (Shephard, 1983). The physician should provide the patient with the maximum-goal heart rate.

A further guide to minimum intensity is that the exercise should cause sweating. The maximum level is indicated by the breathing pattern. Anaerobic work starts at 70–75% of maximum oxygen intake. The build up of lactate in the blood soon leads to vigorous hyperventilation that makes it difficult to talk. If conversation is impossible, the patient is exercising too hard.

Patients may need to moderately increase their exercise intensity every 3–6 weeks to keep improving. Improvement takes several months to years in some persons. Conversely, if the patient stops exercising, deconditioning occurs rapidly. Patients who stop exercising, even for a week, should begin at a lower level when they start exercising again.

Some types of exercise that can be helpful include walk-jog programs, walking programs, or jogging. Walking and then jogging is appropriate for most patients of all ages. By alternating walking with jogging, the patient can vary exercise, distribute periods of different degrees of physical stress over a span of time, and avoid physical stress and boredom. After a period of warming up, the patient starts by jogging for 30 sec, walking for 30 sec, then jogging, then walking. Gradually, patients build up to until they are jogging for 20 min, then walking for 3 min through two complete sets. If patients feel fatigued, breathless, or faint, they should go back to the previous level for 3–5 days before trying to increase to the next level.

Walking is an excellent and safe exercise for all age groups and can be tailored to individual differences and to a wide range of fitness levels. Walking is indeed the exercise of choice for most people. Even though it may seem to be completely safe, except for a sprained ankle occasionally, patients should be warned to stop brisk walking at any point when they experience chest pain or discomfort. If this occurs, they should contact their personal physician.

Because fewer calories are used in walking than in jogging, patients must remember to walk briskly twice as long as they would jog to achieve similar levels of cardiovascular conditioning. An adult male burns the equivalent of 3,500 calories, or 1 lb of fat, in 12 hr of brisk walking. The number of calories burned depends on a number of factors, including body weight and walking rate. Heavier individuals burn more calories than those of lighter weight. Some of the benefits of walking include decreasing the percentage of body fat, improving overall circulation, increasing muscle tone in the legs, and decreasing constipation.

Jogging allows a patient to reach target heart rates more rapidly than walking-jogging or walking alone. However, jogging also is more physically demanding than the other exercises and can lead to physical injuries, particularly to the knees and lower legs if it is attempted too early in the exercise program. In the beginning, continuous jogging should not be done longer than 20 min, and then patients should check their pulse every 5 min. After 10–14 days of jogging continuously for 20 min each day, patients can increase their jogging time to 30 min. If this can be tolerated well for 2

weeks, the jogging period can be increased to 35 or 40 min.

Many people who jog report feeling euphoric, with heightened inner awareness and increased feelings of self-control. Hundreds of excellent books have been written on the benefits of jogging. Two comprehensive books on the subject are George Sheehan's *Medical Advice for Runners* (World Publications) and R. J. Geline's *The Practical Runner* (Collier Books).

Cooling-down period. Any of the exercises mentioned in the preceeding stretching or warm-up sections can be used for cooling-down as well. Cooling-down should take 5–10 min. If exercise is halted too quickly, there is a sudden fall in blood pressure, which can lead to abnormal heart rhythms or, in extreme cases, to loss of consciousness. Hot showers right after exercise can also cause vasodilation and hypotension and should be avoided. Cooling down enables the body to eliminate waste products from the active muscles, which will help eliminate some of the muscle stiffness so common the day after exercise begins.

Helping patients stick with exercise programs. There are a number of strategies that a nurse can use to help patients stick with an exercise program. Setting short- and long-term goals and checking back with the patient to see that he or she has met them is one approach. Another is to have patients record their progress as they go along. The nurse can also help patients choose the best time of day for exercise, one that fits with their personality and lifestyle, and to establish a regular pattern. The idea is to help patients make exercise a habit. Patients can also find a specific place to exercise, dress in clothing that is appropriate for exercising, and think the part by concentrating on bodily movements during exercise. This provides biopsychologic feedback, which is an important part of endurance exercise (Pender, 1987).

Exercise can also become more enjoyable if it

is shared with friends or family members, and if an enjoyable route or setting is selected. Many patients also do well if they can schedule "hard" and "easy" days. An easy day might include warming-up, stretching, and walking for 20 min, or warming-up, stretching, and walking-jogging for 15 min. That is, they choose more vigorous exercise for one day, followed by a more relaxed exercise the next day.

One researcher has suggested four approaches for helping patients stick with exercise and physical conditioning programs: intent, regularity, limits capacity, and concentration (Eischens, 1979). If patients understand why exercise is important to them personally, the program has a better chance of succeeding. For example, is the overall goal to improve health, lose weight, or decrease the risk of coronary disease? Once patients have established their personal health goals, short- and long-term goals can be set.

Regularity can be promoted by alternating exercise days or by using hard days vs. easy days, as outlined before. Three days a week are a minimum. Ideally, the patient would exercise every day. Each person will discover his or her exercise limits and should be encouraged to work at his or her own pace, not to try to compete with anyone else. Patients will become more aware of personal capacities through exercise, such as increased awareness of breathing, muscle movement, and body temperature. Some nurses have had good success charting changing heart rates, increasing exercise capacity, and other health parameters in a personal-growth notebook that is kept by the patient, with help from the nurse (Pender, 1987).

All these steps may help patients stick with it until exercise becomes as natural as eating or sleeping. The goal is to make exercise, like sensible diet, a lifelong habit. *Table 13* lists 14 methods to promote exercise.

PATIENTS WITH SPECIAL PHYSICAL PROBLEMS

Obese patients, diabetic patients, and those with chronic illnesses need specially designed exercise programs. Most of these patients can participate in some type of exercise program, and most benefit from regular exercise. These patients should begin an exercise program only with their physician's consent and with qualified medical supervision.

Diabetic patients. Exercise has beneficial effects on glucose uptake and reduces the need for insulin, according to David Costill, director of the Human Performance Laboratory at Ball State University (Getchell, 1979). He has noted that a diabetic patient who exercises for 30 min or more each day may require 40% less insulin than an inactive diabetic patient does. Glucose uptake is increased 7–20 times during exercise. Then, when exercise stops, the blood flow to the muscles deceases, but glucose uptake remains times that of resting levels for up to an hour (Cantu, 1980). During exercise, insulin levels decrease while muscle intake of glucose increases. This seems to indicate that the muscles can take glucose from the bloodstream during exercise without requiring insulin. Exercise also not only burns calories but also lowers blood glucose levels without insulin. An insulin-dependent diabetic patient risks hypoglycemia if she or he does not decrease intake of insulin or increase intake of carbohydrates before undertaking strenuous exercise (Cantu, 1980). Therefore diabetic patients who exercise should be encouraged to monitor their blood sugar levels after exercise and carry a source of quick-acting glucose if needed.

Exercise is also beneficial to the vascular system and helps retard vascular complications. When there are no special limitations to exercise, nurses can help diabetic patients by stressing a few of the following precautions. First, closed-toe shoes and

Table 13

Methods to Promote Exercise

1. Involve patients in the planning process.

2. Select activities that have already been mastered.

3. Fit the exercise program into the patient's present lifestyle.

4. Plan the exercise at the same time everyday to establish a routine.

5. Develop realistic, achievable goals.

6. Establish rewards.

7. Encourage and reinforce.

8. Teach self-management.

9. Acknowledge the disadvantages of exercise.

10. Use exercise as a social time.

11. Integrate music into the exercise program.

12. Enlist support of companies or community organizations.

13. Serve as a role model to patients.

14. Offer role models to patients.

Source: Extracted from *Community Health Nursing: Process and Practice for Promoting Health,*
3rd Ed., Stanhope, M., Lancaster, J. Mosby Year Book, St. Louis, 1992, p. 605.

socks without wrinkles are a must to avoid trauma to the feet. As mentioned before, diabetic patients should make sure they ingest a controlled amount of carbohydrates before starting exercise to avoid hypoglycemia. Diabetic patients may have to take more gradual steps in the conditioning program, in case they have preexisting cardiac problems. They should also avoid becoming overly fatigued.

Obese patients. Increased body weight increases the stress on the heart, muscles, and joints. Obese persons may also be less flexible and less mobile than those of lower body weight. Some hospital-based exercise programs designed for obese patients have been extremely successful. One of these is the Sittercise program offered at Johns Hopkins University Medical Center (Simonson & Heilman, 1983). Patients exercise while seated in an armless chair, then add a 5-min

walk every day. They are advised against participating in more vigorous exercises in the beginning, such as jogging, jumping rope, climbing stairs, lifting weights, or competitive sports, all of which can be harmful to them.

After 3 months of sittercises and walking, they advance to swimming (a particularly beneficial exercise, because water provides buoyancy and support), more vigorous walking, or exercises on a stationary bicycle. They can then start a program of exercises on a minitrampoline.

In general, correct breathing should be stressed to help maximize ventilatory efficiency during exercise. Warming-up exercises should be selected that can be done while the patient sits in a chair or stands, because floor exercises may be uncomfortable or impossible to do.

Compliance can be improved by planning exercises carefully. The short- and long-term goals of exercise should be determined by the patient in order to provide continuing motivation toward physical fitness over an extended period. Setting realistic goals and using careful reinforcement helps obese patients stay with programs that may at first be uncomfortable and awkward.

Patients with limited mobility. Chronically ill patients with limited mobility or decreased tolerance to exercise, such as those with Parkinson's disease, paralysis, or chronic obstructive pulmonary disease, need an exercise prescription tailored to their specific needs and abilities. All patients, even those with physical limitations, need regular, continuing exercise. For people with physical disabilities, the use of active exercise should be promoted as much as possible (Pender, 1987).

Passive range-of-motion exercises can be used when active range of motion is impossible. Active exercise of nonaffected parts of the body help the patient maintain muscle tone, coordination, and flexibility. Passive range-of-motion exercises can help joints remain mobile and prevent muscle atrophy.

The full scope of exercise planning for chronically ill patients can be found in many excellent texts. Here are a few general guidelines (Pender, 1987):

1. Start physical activity programs gradually, because these patients tire easily.

2. Teach patients relaxation skills, to help them reduce tension or anxiety during exercise.

3. Avoid excessive force against the joints or muscles during exercise.

4. Help patients with feedback during exercise so that they can learn the correct sequence of movements.

5. Help patients keep good posture and keep their bodies aligned during exercise.

6. Perhaps most important, give patients positive reinforcement to encourage them to persist despite difficulties and often-slow progress.

INTERVENING AGAINST STRESS

Programs to reduce stress are in the evolutionary stage. Little concrete information is available about the success of different approaches to intercept and relieve stress. The importance of reducing stress to lessen the risk of CHD is, however, well established (Rosenman & Chesney, 1983). The sympathetic adrenal responses to perceived stress include dilatation of the bronchi, increases in cardiac output and blood volume, dilatation of coronary vessels, enhanced myocardial contractility, and increased heart rate.

Myocardial sensitization causes blood pressure to rise; increases the blood supply to the brain, heart, and skeletal muscles; reduces peristalsis; increases the metabolic rate; enhances blood clotting; and increases aldosterone secretion, which leads to sodium retention and potassium secretion.

Most approaches to treating high levels of stress focus on the three interacting factors in type A behavior, namely, the demands of the environment; the individual's perception of these demands as challenges; and the individual's challenge-prompted responses of time urgency, hostility, aggressiveness, and excess adrenergic arousal. Type A persons have a sense of time urgency and are impatient, demanding, and goal oriented. Type B persons are seen as easygoing, and type C persons seem to thrive on stressful situations.

Many type A behavior patterns are considered strengths and are rewarded in many occupations of the Western world (Rosenman & Chesney, 1983). Thus, it is often difficult for a health care professional to convince type A persons to make far-reaching changes in their social or cultural environment. Instead, the emphasis is placed on helping type A persons recognize the stressful elements that they can control and then recommending changes. Thus, a harried worker facing a large and important project could effectively cope by planning a measured approach to the individual tasks involved and expending physical effort on those tasks.

Using change avoidance, time blocking, and time management techniques, patients can help reduce stress in their environment. An example of change avoidance would be avoiding a stressful job change at a time when a family member is seriously ill. In addition, patients are advised to avoid making lifestyle changes that they might perceive as negative. In addition, such changes should be ones that are seen as challenges rather than threats. For example, learning to play tennis, to swim, or to dance may be an enjoyable challenge to counteract stress.

Time blocking involves setting a specific time aside to adapt to various stressors. Such a block of time may be set aside daily, weekly, or monthly and offers patients time to focus on a specific change and to develop some strategies for adjusting to that change.

For the type A person, time management principles can be used to break tasks into smaller parts so that the entire task does not seem like an impossible chore. Patients are also encouraged to avoid overloading themselves with too many tasks by delegating some tasks to others. Conversely, periods of low stimulation, which can produce negative tension, can also be anticipated and avoided with good time management. A good example of this would be salespersons who spend a lot of time driving between sales calls, time they ordinarily would find extremely boring. They can make this time more stimulating by listening to audiotapes, which may stimulate new ideas or help them develop new skills.

Type A persons can also be helped to adopt a new perspective that can counter their belief that type A behavior has been largely successful for their accomplishments. They must counteract the belief that decreasing the pace of activity, sense of urgency, and competition leads to less productive work and diminished achievement. Instead, patients should be encouraged to pace themselves, work on one task at a time, and approach work in a more relaxed manner. While trying to modify the patient's perceptions the health care team should recognize that the object is not to change a type A person into a type B person but to reduce the typically excessive and probably harmful type A response.

Relaxation techniques. The third approach used to change type A behavior is to alter a person's response to stress and to reduce autonomic

hyperresponsiveness by using techniques such as deep muscle relaxation, meditation, biofeedback, anxiety-management training, and stress-management training. These approaches attempt to minimize the frequency of stress-inducing situations.

Relaxation is thought to decrease the body's oxygen consumption, lower the metabolism, decrease the respiration rate, decrease the heart rate, decrease muscle tension, and decrease systolic and diastolic blood pressure; in short, to counteract the many physiologic responses mentioned at the beginning of this section.

There are many relaxation techniques, most of which involve reclining in a quiet, soundproof room, where light is kept at a low level. The patient is urged to wear loose clothing, to remove shoes and glasses, for example, and to relax in a reclining chair or lounge chair. Patients focus on their own breathing, as they slowly inhale and exhale. The purpose of this is to help increase self-awareness. Patients also use tension-relaxation of their muscles, much as in a yoga class, in which groups of muscles are tightened, held for a short period, then relaxed. Later, patients learn to use imagery and recall to relax. Relaxation through imagery involves concentrating on pleasant scenes or experiences from the past to help feel relaxation. Some scenes might be recalling the warmth of the sun, the feeling of warm sand, the sensation of a gentle breeze, palm trees gently swaying.

Biofeedback has been an important method for managing stress. The foundations of biofeedback depend on a simple idea: People need information about what is going on inside their bodies, because bodily functions cannot be controlled unless information about the functions is available. Some of the physiologic parameters that subjects have been able to control through biofeedback include acceleration and deceleration of heart rate, systolic and diastolic blood pressure, occurrences of PVCs, and alpha-wave activity (recorded on the electroen-

Table 14
Some Options for Stress Management

Task/time Management

Delegate tasks; get help.

Clarify, revise goals and expectations.

Change control/participation expectations or situation.

Provide or obtain information.

Get assertiveness training.

Guard personal freedoms.

Rehearse alternatives.

Learn specific, task-related skills, such as speed-reading, effective writing.

Lifestyle Practices

Optimize aerobic exercise, especially vigorous walking.

Optimize rest.

Use stretching exercises, yoga postures.

Use humor.

Decrease intake of caffeine and nicotine.

Decrease intake of alcohol, sedatives, and recreational drugs.

Eat fewer simple carbohydrates; increase complex carbohydrates.

Eat fewer saturated fats; eat more polyunsaturated fats.

Relaxation Techniques

Learn the relaxation response.

Learn progressive relaxation.

Use autogenic training.

Use creative visualization.

Use the quieting response.

Try transcendental meditation, yoga.

Source: Harris, J. S., & Hastings, J. E. (1987). *The Preventive Approach to Patient Care* (p. 370). New York: Elsvier.

and to function effectively to modify the fight-or-flight (stress) response.

Ray Rosenman, who was one of the first physicians to recognize the type A personality, suggests several methods that have been successful for helping patients change their responses to challenge or stress:

1. *Self-observation.* Type A patients, who typically are not aware of their compulsive or obsessive behavior, are asked to observe and keep a record of daily actions that arouse a sense of time urgency, competition, hostility, or other type A responses.

2. *Self-contracting.* Type A patients are helped to write personal contracts to modify defined, specific type A behavior on specified occasions.

3. *Modeling.* Physicians demonstrate attempts at controlling their own behavior and, by so doing, serve as models for patients who are trying to change their own type A behavior.

4. *Referral.* Patients are referred to therapists familiar with behavior modification and type A behavior.

Table 14 lists several stress-management options. In some cases, the nurse can help patients work on strategies to reduce stresses in their environment, or patients may be referred to special stress-management programs.

Dr. Rosenman offers a number of drills, or exercises for type A individuals, including drills against "hurry sickness," hostility, and a category called "things worth being." The following are examples of some of the strategies type A persons can use to avoid stress (Friedman & Rosenman, 1974).

cephalogram). During the training period, instruments help patients learn to read and interpret body signals. However, after the training period, patients must learn to do this without the help of equipment

As a drill against the sense of time urgency, or hurry sickness:

1. One of the most important new habits you can establish is to review at least once a week the original causes of your present hurry sickness. Just as a doctor is far more likely to be able to cure a disease if he or she knows what causes it, you, too, will be better prepared to alter your sense or urgency if you know why you have it.

2. Every morning, noon, and midafternoon, remind yourself, preferably while looking in the mirror, that life is always unfinished. We suggest this because often type A individuals doggedly persist in believing that they can finish all the events of their life at the end of every day. Actually, they can do so only by bullet, poison, or a jump from a high building or bridge. You are only finished when you are dead.

3. Never forget, when confronted by any task, to ask yourself the following questions: (a) Will this matter have importance 5 years from now? and (b) Must I do this right now, or do I have enough time to think about the best way to accomplish it?

4. Tell yourself at least once a day that no enterprise ever failed because it was executed too slowly, too well.

5. With a companion, purposely go to restaurants and theaters where you know you will have to wait. If your companion is your spouse, remember that you spend far longer periods alone with her or him in your own home without fidgeting.

Some examples of a drill against hostility include the following:

1. If you are overtly hostile, remind yourself that you are hostile. Being forewarned, you are far less inclined to flare up at any stimulus short of one that would induce hostility in anyone.

2. Begin to express your thanks or appreciation to others when they have performed services for you. And do not do so, like so many hostile type A individuals, with merely a grunt of thanks. Take the time to look the man or woman who has served you well full in the face and then in full and gracious sentences let him or her know how grateful you are.

3. Begin to smile at as many people as often as you can. Begin this regularly and frequently with the people you may meet in corridors and elevators of your building. Then begin to smile at persons whom you may encounter while walking in a city square or park or in your own neighborhood. While this may seem to be quite contrived and hypocritical, that will be true only if you fail to find the qualities in other people that might command your respect, admiration, or affection.

Many books and educational materials are available that delve deeply into the relationship between stress and increased risk of disease, particularly CHD. One good source, which discusses the role of stress in hypertension and CHD is *Stress, Health, and the Social Environment,* by J. P. Henry and P. M. Stevens (New York, Springer-Verlag, 1977).

PATIENTS RECOVERING FROM MYOCARDIAL INFRACTION

Patients recovering from an MI can benefit from all the programs discussed thus far: stress reduction, weight loss, and lowering plasma glucose and cholesterol levels. Most of the programs that can be offered to all patients, with the exception of exercise programs, are also helpful to patients who have had an MI. Some need specialized exercise programs.

The major benefit from an exercise program

after a serious cardiac event such as an MI or coronary artery bypass grafting is improvement in functional capacity. This includes an increase in maximal cardiac output and oxygen consumption, decrease in the resting heart rate, and more rapid return to normal heart rate after exercise.

Studies are under way to see if exercise training changes myocardial ischemia or myocardial function in humans. There is some suggestion that long-term physical activity does increase coronary vascularity and thus improve myocardial perfusion and function; however, it still is not known if this occurs in humans, particularly older patients who have significant degrees of atherosclerosis (Chung, 1986).

Prolonged bed rest and lack of ambulation lead to a number of physiologic losses (Wenger, 1985). Prolonged bed rest decreases physical work capacity 20– 25% after only 3 weeks of immobilization. In addition, after only 7–10 days of bed rest, circulating blood volume drops 700–800 ml. Blood viscosity increases because of greater contraction of the plasma volume than of the red cell mass, increasing the risk of thromboembolism. Muscle contractile strength deceases by 10–15% within the first week of bed rest.

Lack of exercise after an MI can also produce a number of psychological problems. Anxiety and depression, which offer occur after an MI, may be increased by lack of exercise. Anxiety reflects the realistic fear of dying, and depression is related to the fear of inability to return to work, to normal sexual function, and to a previous lifestyle. In contrast, patients who exercise tend to feel better; have more confidence and higher self-esteem; and show less anxiety, depression, denial, and dependency. They also seem better able to face life crises. Exercise also helps patients renounce the "sick role" and get back to their previous lifestyle.

Candidates for exercise programs. Before beginning an exercise program, patients are usually tested in the hospital with an exercise stress test or bicycle ergometer test. With these methods, physicians can detect ischemia not evident during rest (ST segment depression), measure the heart rate during activity, and diagnose arrhythmias or conduction defects (Pender, 1987).

Patients who are good candidates for an exercise program generally have had an uncomplicated clinical course. Good candidates tend to be younger and have not had previous infractions (Wenger, 1983).

Contraindications to starting a patient on an exercise regimen after an MI, include the following:

* Heart muscle damaged to extent of aneurysm or weakness in the heart muscle wall

* Acute heart failure

* Myocarditis

* Grossly irregular heart beats (multifocal ectopic arrhythmias)

* Progressive or sudden onset of severe chest pain on exertion

* Some forms of congenital or valvular heart disease

* Recurrent pulmonary embolism or thrombophlebitis

* Complete heart block

Exercise usually begins while the patient is still in the cardiac care unit, where he or she can be supervised by health care professionals who can assess the patient's response (heart rate and blood pressure) to activity. This is also a protective setting where any problems can be taken care of immediately.

Patients can begin low-level activity in the first few days after an infarction. Those with complications can begin gradual ambulation once such problems are controlled. Most units allow patients to participate in low-intensity activities, such as those requiring about 1–2 METS. Self-care activities can fulfill these requirements, for example, feeding oneself, taking care of personal needs, using a bedside commode, and sitting in a bedside chair. Patients can participate unless the following signs or symptoms occur: chest pain, dyspnea, palpitations, heart rate greater than 120 beats per minute, ST segment changes on the ECG, or a fall of more than 10–15 mm Hg in systolic blood pressure. If any of these occur, activity is suspended, and patients rest.

During the remainder of the hospitalization, gradually increasing exercise is encouraged so that the patient can perform typical homebound activities after discharge. Typically, discharge occurs 7–14 days after an infarction with an uncomplicated hospital course. Patients perform personal care; sit in a chair for increasing periods; and perform supervised selected dynamic warm-up exercises that use their arms, legs, and trunk. Walking is another important component of the in-hospital program, with the pace and length gradually increased. If patients must climb stairs at home, they are encouraged to use stair climbing while in the hospital.

Patients may at first be afraid to start an exercise program soon after an MI, but their safety has been reported in a large number of studies (Wenger, 1985). Patients can be reassured by learning that exercise does not increase the incidence of angina pectoris, reinfarction, arrhythmias, heart failure, ventricular aneurysm, cardiac rupture, or sudden cardiac death. A gradual exercise program allays such fears. Once patients see that they are safe and no calamity befalls them, they will be much better prepared for discharge home.

After a patient has recovered and has enough endurance to return to work (usually 4–8 weeks after the infarction), more intensive exercise training, with the goal of enhancing cardiovascular function, is appropriate. It is recommended that patients be tested while they are using their pre-

scribed medications. This may include ß-adrenergic blockers, calcium channel blockers, digitalis, diuretics, and antihypertensive drugs (Chung, 1986).

A typical exercise prescription. In most exercise programs for patients recovering from an infraction, patients exercise at least two or three times a week, usually not on successive days. More exercise is not necessarily better. More than four exercise sessions a week does not improve the maximal oxygen uptake of most middle-aged adults (Chung, 1986). Patients who are not very fit and sedentary elderly patients can improve their physical work capacity by using as few as one or two exercise sessions a week.

Most exercise sessions should last 30–45 min, including warming-up and cooling-down periods. Patients should attain a heart rate that is 70–85% of the highest level safely reached on ECG stress testing. This level corresponds to 60–78% of the peak oxygen uptake, an effective but safe range within which to stimulate aerobic metabolism. A lower range, 70–75%, is recommended for those who exercise at home or alone in an unsupervised setting. Higher target rates, such as 80–85%, are advisable for those who will be exercising in a supervised hospital or outpatient program (Chung, 1986).

Exercise programs are always tailored to the individual, because the needs and goals, the degree of fitness, the type of cardiovascular impairment, and personal likes and dislikes vary greatly from person to person. In addition, some patients have excellent access to programs and equipment, whereas others live in remote or rural areas where facilities are limited.

In the beginning, patients recovering from an infraction or other cardiac problems should be encouraged to participate in programs with medical supervision. Patients can get help with unfamiliar exercises and be motivated and reassured that they

Table 15
Warning Signs During Exercise

If any of the following should occur during exercise, the exercise should be stopped, and an overall evaluation of the patient's condition should be made by the cardiac rehabilitation staff or other medical personnel.

Symptoms	Signs	Measurements
Increasing angina	Pallor; cold, moist skin	Excessive rise in blood pressure (diastolic ≥20 mm Hg)
Severe dyspnea	Cyanosis	Sudden fall of blood pressure (≥10 mm Hg)
Severe fatigue	Staggering gait	ST depression >0.2 mV
Claudication pain	Confused response to questioning	More than three in 10 sec
Dizziness or faintness		Other major dysrhythmias

Source: Shephard, R. J. (1983) Exercise and primary prevention of coronary heart disease. In R. N. Podell & M. M. Stewart (Eds.), *Primary Prevention of Coronary Heart Disease* (p. 227). Menlo Park, CA: Addison-Wesley.

are safe, and emergency facilities are available if needed. In most cases, patients are asked to sign consent forms before entering an exercise program. This has obvious medicolegal benefits, but it also gives the health care team the chance to review the reasons for an exercise program, safety tips, warning signs *(Table 15)*, and ways to avert problems. It is also a good time to stress that exercise is only one part of the rehabilitation program, which may also include diet, weight control, stopping smoking, and appropriate ways to take medication.

It is also a good time to warn patients not to exercise when they are unusually tired or under excessive stress. When persons return to an exercise program after stopping exercise for several days or weeks because of an illness or for other reasons, they will have lost ground and will have to start back at a lower level than before. Then they can gradually return to higher levels of exercise. Type A or otherwise very competitive patients should be repeatedly warned about trying to exercise harder than they should.

Just as with all sound exercise programs, programs for patients who have had an MI or bypass surgery include a warm-up and stretching period, a training or endurance component, and a cooling-down period. All three phases are important.

Warm-up. The first 5–10 min of exercise includes primarily stretching, slow walking, and range-of-motion exercises, as well as selected calisthenics. These will enable muscles to warm up and joints to adapt and will also improve the general circulation. This part of the exercise program is particularly important for elderly or previously sedentary people.

Endurance. The next 15–20 min involves aerobic training or endurance, designed to stimulate the transport of oxygen. Usually this segment involves either walk-jog sequences or exercises on a stationary bicycle or a treadmill. These exercises primarily train the leg muscles, so patients will also need arm-training exercises such as calisthenics and the use of shoulder wheels and rowing machines. At first, exercises are low-level and rhythmic.

Patients who will be exercising at home need detailed, specific explanations of each exercise in writing, for example, how many of each type, how long each type should last, and the desirable target heart rate. it is also helpful to describe the best type of clothing to wear and to warn against exercising after meals, in adverse weather, and so forth.

In time, other types of exercises that will use

large muscle groups are added, including rope-jumping, swimming, cycling, rowing, and aerobics. Even though selected games make exercise more fun, in the early days after an infarction, the emphasis should be on quiet, rhythmic exercise. Most cardiac patients use about 50 calories per exercise session, then gradually progress to 200–300 calories per session (Chung, 1986). (A rate of about 300 calories is usually recommended for healthy sedentary patients starting out in an exercise program.)

If patients are not being monitored with continuous ECGs, they should periodically check their heart rate response, to see that it is in the desired range. If heart rate irregularities are noted, the patient should have an ECG rhythm strip recorded.

Interval training is also a helpful approach. This involves alternating periods of activity and rest or of high- and low-intensity activities. By switching from more to less vigorous exercise, patients can have a higher total workload at each session before symptoms, such as angina, appear.

For the first year or so, at least some of the weekly exercise sessions should be carried out under medical supervision, so that the health care team will know how well the patient is responding. Games such as volleyball, basketball, tennis, and handball add variety to the exercise program and help supply exercise to both the upper and lower parts of the body. In most cases, because these are vigorous sports, they are not added to the exercise prescription until later.

Cool-down. The last 10–15 min of exercise involves a gradual decrease in intensity. Many programs use walking or light calisthenics to help the patient cool down. Cooling down allows the heart rate to slowly subside and avoids postexercise hypotension, which can occur when maximum peripheral vasodilation is present, causing pooling of blood in the legs (Chung, 1986).

Patients seem to stay with exercise better when

their spouses and family have a positive attitude toward the exercise program. The goal of long-term physical activity is to help the patient become reasonably independent. This process involves several steps, including initial monitoring; then weaning from monitoring; and moving from a rigidly structured exercise program to a more relaxed one that is pleasurable, convenient, and appropriate for the individual patient. Patients should be encouraged to add exercise to their lives whenever possible, such as walking up stairs rather than using an elevator or walking or riding a bicycle rather than driving short distances.

COMPLICATIONS

If patients do not seem to improve or cannot reach increasing exercise goals, they need reassurance and possibly additional medical and surgical therapy. Not all patients can improve their cardiac function, even with appropriate exercises (Chung, 1986). If function is not improving, the patient may have left ventricular dysfunction or even overt cardiac failure at higher levels of exercise. The underlying CHD may have progressed.

There are general guidelines for helping patients avoid difficulties while exercising (Shephard, 1983). It certainly is better to prevent complications than to have to treat cardiovascular complications from exercise (Shephard, 1983). The guidelines are

1. If the patient shows any adverse reactions to exercise, the exercise prescription should be set at a pulse rate 10 to 15 beats/min below the point where the problem develops.

2. Teach patients to recognize angina and arrhythmias.

3. If the patient is under severe emotional stress or the weather is too hot, too cold, or extremely humid, the exercise prescription should be temporarily reduced.

4. Warming-up and cooling-down periods are important to ease the body into exercise and then to relax it after exercise. These two steps also help prevent orthopedic injuries and musculoskeletal problems.

5. Patients should avoid hot or cold showers after exercise and should not linger in very humid dressing rooms.

6. If the patient has a fever or a viral infection, is very tired, or has systemic signs or symptoms, he or she should avoid vigorous exercise.

7. If a patient feels more than just a little tired the day after exercise, the level may be too high and should be readjusted.

8. People with angina often find that their signs and symptoms are aggravated when they exercise in cold, dry air. This is caused by cutaneous vasoconstriction, which increases the cardiac work rate; in addition, breathing in cold air also induces exercise bronchospasm in persons with sensitive airways. Using a jogging mask in cold weather may help patients avoid such problems.

9. In very hot weather, distance running can cause dehydration and a dangerous rise in body temperature.

10. Advise patients to wear well-cushioned shoes with appropriate inserts or padding to counteract any gait abnormalities.

11. When a patient changes the type of exercise, for example, substitutes tennis for jogging or jumps rope indoors because of icy conditions outside, a different set of muscles is used. The patient should slow activity for a few days until the body adjusts to the new activity.

Any exercise program should be gradually and progressively increased on an individual basis. Some sports are not recommended for older adults (more than 50 years old), especially those who are highly competitive or who have limited functional capacity.

The next chapter examines the ways in which nurses act as health educators, including the challenge of getting adult patients to change long-term harmful behaviors that place the patients at risk of cardiovascular disease.

EXAM QUESTIONS

CHAPTER 7
Questions 68–79

68. Why is it important to evaluate all the medications a hypertensive patient is taking?

    a. To save the patient money by uncovering duplicate agents

    b. To identify certain products that may be contributing to hypertension, such as nonsteroidal antiinflammatory agents

    c. To complete the patient's records

    d. To determine compliance

69. True or false: Most smokers can benefit from one approach, rather than a combination of approaches, to stopping smoking.

    a. True

    b. False

70. Which of the following is an indication to stop exercise?

    a. Decrease in diastolic pressure of more than 75 mm Hg

    b. Increase in heart rate greater than 10% of baseline

    c. Increase in diastolic pressure of more than 20 mm Hg

    d. Decrease in heart rate greater than 10% of baseline

71. The difference between Step-One and Step-Two diets is:

    a. Saturated fatty acids are further reduced in the Step-One diet.

    b. Total fat intake can remain at 50% of calories on the Step-Two diet.

    c. Saturated fatty acids are further reduced in the Step-Two diet.

    d. The Step-One diet is used only for children.

72. Regular vigorous exercise does which of the following?

    a. Decreases blood cell mass and blood volume

    b. Increases blood oxygen levels

    c. Increases serum triglyceride levels

    d. Decreases glucose tolerance

73. Maximum heart rate is usually predicted by using which of the following?

    a. 220 minus age in years

    b. 275 minus age in years

    c. 350 minus age in years

    d. 150 minus age in years

74. True or false: Endurance exercise is vigorous but not excessively strenuous activity that primarily involves the leg muscles.

    a. True

    b. False

75. One strategy nurses can use that will help patients stick with exercise programs is to:

    a. Be firm about insisting patients exercise every day.

    b. Help patients set short- and long-term exercise goals.

    c. Discourage patients from recording their progress at first.

    d. Recommend that patients exercise only in the morning.

76. Which of the following is a major benefits of exercise for a diabetic patient?

    a. It promotes a sense of well-being.

    b. Glucose uptake decreases during exercise.

    c. It reduces the need for insulin.

    d. When exercise ends, glucose levels rapidly fall.

77. Time blocking is which of the following?

    a. A method of ignoring time

    b. A technique used to help type A persons adapt to various stressors

    c. A biofeedback technique

    d. Weight-reduction strategy

78. Prolonged bed rest and lack of ambulation decrease physical work capacity by what percentage after only 3 weeks of immobilization?

    a. 10–15

    b. 5–10

    c. 50

    d. 20–25

79. Which of the following is a contraindication to starting a patient on an exercise regimen after an MI?

    a. Use of ß-blockers

    b. Grossly irregular heart beats

    c. Age above 50 years

    d. None of the above

CHAPTER 8

THE NURSE AS EDUCATOR

CHAPTER OBJECTIVE

After studying this chapter, the reader will have an understanding of the challenges of educating adults about changing behaviors that place them at high risk for heart disease.

LEARNING OBJECTIVES

After studying this chapter, the reader should be able to

1. List at least three characteristics of an adult learner.

2. Outline the five main phases of the nurse-client relationship.

3. List at least three false assumptions about educating patients.

4. Explain how control and learned helplessness affect compliance.

INTRODUCTION

After a long day of seeing and counseling patients, many of whom have not followed instructions, a nurse may feel that much of the effort to help patients change harmful behavior has been futile.

A physician once remarked that he felt he was really practicing suicide prevention instead of med- icine because so many of his patients seemed bent on shortening their lives through heavy smoking, overeating, and lack of exercise. The hypertensive patient who will not take his or her medication and the seriously overweight patient who can not seem to stick with a moderately restricted diet are com- mon examples. How can a nurse reach such patients and have an impact on changing their behavior and helping them adapt a more healthful lifestyle?

This chapter looks at the nurse's role as health educator. It examines some of the barriers a nurse must overcome to reach patients to help them change their lifestyle and to lessen their risk of heart disease.

NURSES AS EDUCATORS

The nurse has a unique opportunity to pro- mote better personal health for patients or clients through expertise and continuing face-to-face contacts with such people. Through personal example and direct teaching efforts, nurses provide important health care information.

Although health care delivery is the central part of nursing, educating patients about their health is also a major responsibility for most nurses. In fact, as Ruth Beckmann Murray, Assistant Dean of the School of Nursing at St. Louis University, has noted, a staff nurse or a private care nurse may be more of a teacher than someone who is officially identified as a "teacher" (Murray & Zentner, 1985). A history teacher may teach high school students from 9 a.m. to 3 p.m., 5 days a week, but a nurse can spend nearly every waking moment teaching.

Nurses teach through example, beginning at home by teaching their family members about health. This might be exemplified by noticing early signs or symptoms of diabetes in a father and sending him to an internist for tests. Or, this could be manifested as the first aid given to a son who fractures his arm. A nurse is also a teacher when friends and neighbors ask questions about vitamins or about products that purportedly reverse the aging process, a miracle cure for baldness, a pill that makes pounds melt away overnight, or the side effects of a new drug.

Dr. Murray adds that nurses teach no matter what professional position they hold. She notes:

> The staff nurse can teach while giving the patient a bath. The nurse in the doctor's office or clinic can do spot teaching while preparing a patient for examination. The public health nurse or visiting nurse can teach while working with specific situations in the home. The industrial nurse can teach while taking down information about workers. Of course, the nurse is also a teacher while instructing students, but teaching is more basic than a professional job. Also, your teaching is not limited to the task at hand. One industrial nurse in a two-week period encountered 40 problems offered by the employees that were unrelated to their treatments. Most problems concerned health care needs of family members.

There are ever-increasing opportunities to teach health in the community. Hospitals and community health clinics, community health programs, senior citizen centers, and residential day-care centers offer programs aimed at improving health care and preventing disease. Schools provide yet another setting and often invite nurses and other health care professionals to give programs on basic health care. Even businesses are offering employees health-oriented programs, including hypertension and cholesterol screening.

Medical group practices are developing relationships with professional nurses to expand services to consumers (Pender, 1987). Nurse-educators may have baccalaureate, master's, doctoral, or nurse-practitioner degrees. They are responsible for assessing, teaching, counseling, and providing direct care to clients. In these settings, they often perform risk appraisals, provide health education and nutrition counseling, teach stress-management techniques, counsel patients about human sexuality, and suggest lifestyle modifications. Health maintenance organizations place particular emphasis on prevention and health promotion and cannot fulfill their legal purpose unless they use the talents of a wide range of people, including professional nurses.

Two other settings should also be mentioned, group and independent nursing practices. In ever-increasing numbers, nurses are setting up group practices and contracting to offer services to hospitals, large groups of physicians, schools, businesses, and industries. Nurses who offer private services as health consultants and teachers contract to teach on a long- or a short-term basis and may provide the same types of services mentioned earlier.

CHOOSING TEACHING STRATEGIES

Teaching conjures up many images, most based on personal experiences as students. Because of childhood experiences, most people have preconceived notions of what teaching-learning situations should be like (Rorden, 1987). One is the relative formality in which teaching-learning is conducted; the second is the structure that ought to be used to guide the interaction of the teacher and the learner.

Formality is the psychosocial distance between teacher and learner. The more formal the setting, the more obvious is the role of the teacher as the "expert" and the greater his or her sense of control. Generally, teachers who are relatively inexperienced or lack confidence presenting material tend to prefer a more formal teacher-student relationship. The structure is the setting and progression of learning.

Educating patients involves influencing behavior, producing changes in knowledge and attitudes, and introducing skills that are needed to maintain and improve health. Although the process begins with information, it includes interpretation and integration of the information in such a way as to help change attitudes or behavior to improve the patient's health status.

These changes occur over time and involve ongoing reassessment of patients' level of knowledge, attitudes, and skills, as well as evaluation of their motivation to make sometimes enormous changes in lifestyle and behaviors. This translates to tailoring education to individual patients, considering their strengths and weaknesses, and, most important, knowing how to help adults learn. Unfortunately, too often adults are taught as though they were children. For many adults, too, the thought of "health education" conjures up visions of sitting in a fifth-grade classroom while a formal lesson is presented.

In addition, many health care professionals are better at prescribing health care changes than at motivating their patients to adopt more healthful ways of life. Change is the result of a lengthy process and may take years of repeated effort and frustration until the right combination of motivating events, spontaneous or premeditated, occurs. A good example of this might be the long-time chain-smoker who has read and discarded all the literature about the medical problems associated with smoking but is finally motivated to stop once and for all when a suspicious spot shows up on his or her chest radiograph.

Ten false assumptions about patient education. In her excellent book, *Issues and Concepts in Patient Education,* Barbara Klug Redman, Professor of Nursing at the University of Colorado, lists 10 false assumptions about educating patients that are worth considering:

1. A patient learns what he or she has been told.

2. Learning in health environments occurs exclusively or primarily when the patient is being "taught," usually in a formal setting like a class.

3. Knowledge about a disease significantly affects the patient's compliance with the treatment regimen for that disease.

4. Knowing "why" is necessary for knowing "how."

5. Helping a patient learn how to carry out the desired behavior or altering the environment by changing clinic schedules to shorten waiting time is not an educational intervention.

6. Until a patient is ready, he or she will not learn.

7. Attitudes have to be changed before behavior will change.

8. A written plan of teaching intervention resembles what occurs.

9. Once patients have learned the "basics" about a health condition or a behavior they are to perform, they generally need little additional education and what they do require they can usually obtain by themselves.

10. Physical care always has a higher priority than educating patients does.

Teaching materials. Selecting good teaching materials is important. In many cases, the first educational effort is verbal, with advice given on a one-to-one basis. Many physicians use this approach. However, studies have shown that much of the message delivered in this way is not retained by patients and vanishes as soon as they leave the waiting room. If the educational effort is limited to a one-time personal message, there is little chance that the behavior will change or that goals will be achieved. Instead, the message must be repeated again and again and be supplemented by other teaching strategies, including enlisting the help of the patient's families.

When selecting a teaching style that is acceptable to the patient, a nurse can be guided by the tone and nature of interactions that precede the planned teaching session and by verbal and nonverbal responses from the patient as teaching begins (Rorden, 1987). This starts with the first contact. In a way, the nurse is making an "educational diagnosis" at first contact, just as a nursing diagnosis was made at an earlier point. When assessing the educational needs of a patient, there are several questions to ask. What information does the patient need? What attitudes need to be explored? What skills does this patient need to perform health care behaviors? What factors in the patient's environment are barriers to successfully changing behaviors or learning new skills?

Sometimes, of course, the pressures of time, interruptions from other patients, emergencies, distractions, and lack of privacy can interrupt the most thoroughly prepared lesson plans and can interfere with patient-nurse communication. It is helpful to carefully assess the learning environment before teaching begins. For example, if the patient can not be moved from a noisy area full of distractions, the nurse might pull the curtains, adjust the light, and have written materials the patient can study. The challenge is to make the setting as conducive to learning as possible.

Limitations of time may also interfere with an ideal educational setting. The nurse may have only a short time to help the patient prepare for a procedure that is scheduled to begin immediately. By evaluating how much time may be needed to help the patient learn about a certain procedure or self-care approach, the nurse can plan for other teaching materials, such as a videotape, or even ask other professionals with expertise in that area to help.

Remember, too, that education of patients often takes place in a stressful setting, such as in the cardiac care unit. If a patient can participate in discussion or other types of activities, the quality of learning improves, and the patient may be able to better focus attention on goals for the future.

PHASES OF A NURSE-CLIENT EDUCATIONAL RELATIONSHIP

Regardless of the setting and arrangements, the nurse-client relationship progresses through a number of phases, beginning with the first contact and continuing through termination and follow-up. Remember that the teaching relationship is a helping relationship rather than a social relationship, which is much more familiar to the patient. The relationship can generally be divided into five phases: (a) the initial phase, (b) a transition phase, (c) a working phase, (d) a termination phase, and (e) a follow-up phase (Pender, 1987).

Initial phase. The initial phase starts with the first contact. This is an excellent time to learn as much as possible about the client and the areas where help is needed. Mutual understanding of the client's health goals and expectations can also be explored. The learning orientation must be to sustain and enhance the independence of the patient, while helping him or her develop self-care competency. This phase also works as a two-way process, allowing the patient to assess the nurse as a professional and to judge the nurse's professionalism, expertise, trustworthiness, reliability, and helpfulness (Smitherman, 1981).

When selecting a teaching style that is acceptable to the patient, a nurse can be guided by the tone and nature of interactions that precede the planned teaching and by verbal and nonverbal responses from the patient as teaching begins (Rorden, 1987).

Getting to know the patient and the people who are important to him or her gives the nurse the best chance to clearly and specifically determine the patient's learning needs. Establishing rapport at the first meeting lays the groundwork for good communication between patient and nurse. This involves considering the patient's background, educational level, and ability to communicate. What about the patient who can not speak or comprehend English, or who knows only a smattering of English? In most larger hospitals and clinics, a member of the staff will be available to translate for non–English-speaking patients, and professional translators are available in the community. Also, a member of the patient's family may be able to help. In most families, at least one member can speak and understand English. Such a person can be very helpful when the diagnosis is discussed and during later efforts at education.

Deciding where to begin can also pose a dilemma, particularly when the client needs to know about a variety of different health behaviors. Two criteria have been suggested for determining where to start (Pender, 1987):

1. Start with the area that is most important to the client at the time.

2. Start with the area of knowledge that will contribute most to maintaining or enhancing health.

Patients do have definite ideas about what they want to know and what is most important to them. Unfortunately, sometimes their interest is not the area that poses the greatest threat to them. An over-

weight smoker, for example, may want to lose weight for cosmetic reasons, overlooking his or her chronic bronchitis. Or, the chain-smoker may want to start a good exercise program. In the latter case, a physically active smoker is obviously an improvement over a sedentary smoker, and the patient may also eventually become aware that smoking cuts down on lung capacity and physical endurance. At that point, the patient may also become interested in stopping smoking. This case also illustrates an important point in the nurse-patient relationship: The teaching priorities should be those of the patient, not the nurse. Starting where the patient's greatest interest is lets the nurse gain control over health education interactions, enhancing their meaningfulness to the patient (Pender, 1987).

In the first phase of the relationship, the nurse can help the patient make informed choices about health protection and promotion, through health assessment, clarification of values, and self-care education. The information from the health history, family health history, and specialized questionnaires such as those discussed earlier can be helpful here.

Transition phase. The second major phase is the transition phase. With time, the patient's initial enthusiasm may wane or fluctuate; he or she may be enthusiastic and then apathetic and may accept or reject some health care suggestions. This can be especially true of patients who have low self-esteem or who have difficulty establishing close relationships with other people. Here it may be helpful to try to understand the patient's point of view even more thoroughly by asking such questions as "How do you view yourself and your significance to others?" or "What are your major ambitions or goals?"

Working phase. The third phase is the working phase, one of the action portions of the learning process. Once health goals are determined, both the nurse and the client can work closely, using regularly scheduled visits to allow the client to put into action various alternatives and then to evaluate their success. The support of the spouse and other family members is particularly important during this time, because no major change in attitude or lifestyle is ever easy. The types of programs implemented in the working phase include physical fitness programs, nutrition programs, weight control programs, reduction and management of stress, and development of meaningful social support systems (Pender, 1987).

Termination phase. The fourth phase is the termination phase, in which regular contacts are gradually tapered, then ended, and the client assumes responsibility for continuing the health care changes made during the earlier phases. This can sometimes be a difficult phase. However, it can be made easier for everyone if the objectives and the length of time required to accomplish them are spelled out clearly at the outset. For example, the nurse can tell the client at an early meeting that the training takes about 12 weeks and then appointments taper off during the following 6 months. The impact of termination can also be lessened if the family is given an ever-increasing role and participation in prevention and health promotion.

During the termination phase, a helpful strategy is to involve clients in assessing the progress that has been made and to help them develop plans for self-care, while stressing that future contact is always an option. The ultimate goal is, of course, to help clients manage their own health and lives

---

Table 16
Steps in a Lesson Sequence

Beginning
1. Confirm the patient's knowledge base and motivation.
2. Get the patient's attention.
3. Clarify the objectives and present "organizer."

Middle
4. Present the content of the lesson; get feedback.
5. Provide an example.

End
6. Reinforce learning.
7. Summarize and evaluate learning.

Source: Rorden, J. E. (1987). *Nurses as health teachers: A practical guide.* Philadelphia: Saunders.

---

more successfully.

Follow-up phase. The final phase is follow-up with periodic contacts. These meetings can reinforce the progress made by the patient or can provide refresher sessions. Visits every 6 months or at other appropriate intervals can help reinforce the behavioral changes the patient has learned. Follow-up can involve repeat appointments in the clinical setting or home visits or letter or telephone follow-up. Face-to-face contact is preferable for nurse and client to discuss any new problems or difficulties that may have arisen since the last contact (Pender, 1987). The follow-up phase thus allows the nurse to work with new clients, while keeping open the possibility that former clients can have active help if needed.

STEPS IN A LESSON SEQUENCE

There are many different approaches to lesson planning, and many excellent nursing education texts can provide in-depth guidelines for this. This book does not go into great detail but briefly outlines one example suggested by Judith Waring Rorden, director of Koala Associates, in San Jose, CA. Dr. Rorden suggests dividing the lesson sequence into three major parts–beginning, middle, and end—and offers seven steps from start to finish *(Table 16)*.

The first step is to confirm the patient's knowledge of the subject and his or her reasons for wanting to change some or several parts of his or her lifestyle. Doing this will let the nurse know where to start. Otherwise, the nurse may be wasting time with an approach that is too advanced or too limited for the particular patient. Or, the nurse may target an area the patient has no interest in or rejects.

Each person comes to the sessions with a different level and background of health information. For example, one patient may be knowledgeable about diet or about cardiovascular risks, whereas another may be puzzled by even elementary medical terms such as hypertension or angina. One way to approach this is to simply ask the patient what his or her experience has been or what he or she knows about heart disease in general.

At this early stage, it is important to consider patients' perception of their health needs and their own situation. The following example is an extreme one, but it helps to underline the importance of understanding the patient's real-life situation when teaching and making lifestyle recommendations (Rankin & Duffy, 1983).

Rosie, an obese, 55-year-old patient with adult-onset diabetes and hypertension, had several educational sessions with her physician and two nurses. She showed that she understood her diet and medications and could manage them well at home. However, she did not manage her diabetes at home and was admitted as an emergency patient several times. When the health care team investigated further, they found that she was having marital problems and had a complicated social and financial situation. Her husband was sexually involved with other women, and she felt he should be taking care of her.

At one home visit, the nurse noted that five of Rosie's six children were still living at home (the youngest was 23 years old), and only one of the children was working. The patient's husband worked in a local factory, and their only other income was her disability insurance check. Her

medical care was covered by Medicaid. The family did not have a car and lived in a small, poorly kept, four-room house. Although the health care team felt confident that the patient knew how to manage her health problems at home, it became apparent that many other factors were interfering with her life and influencing her decision not to manage her diabetes. After several more admissions for an MI and a cerebrovascular accident, Rosie died.

Therefore, even the most carefully designed lesson plan will not work unless the nurse first considers the patient's perception of the patient's health needs and assesses the patient's situation at work and at home. Effective education requires an understanding of all the factors that influence a patient every day: values, beliefs, attitudes, current life stresses, religion, and previous experiences with health care and life goals.

Another important point to remember is that providing health information alone is not enough. If health care professionals were asked to define "patient education," they would be likely to say this is handing out information to patients about problems and treatments. A well-equipped file drawer and informative posters in the office may be helpful, but they are not enough.

Too often, when patients fail to assimilate the information or to change harmful behaviors, it is assumed that they were not given enough information or that they did not to comprehend it. Learning information alone does not ensure that behavioral change will follow. One educator asks health care professionals to compare their own behavior with behaviors they prescribe for patients. Although health care professionals may tell patients to refrain from smoking, exercise regularly, fasten their seat belts, keep weight within prescribed limits, and floss every day, how many health professionals comply with all these practices?

The following are a few questions to guide this process:

1. What are the client's most noticeable values?

2. Does the client have any existing health problems that need to be considered when developing a plan for a healthier lifestyle?

3. To what extent does the client believe that he or she can personally control his or her health?

4. What is the nutritional status of the patient?

5. What diseases is the client at risk for?

6. What sources of stress is the client exposed to?

7. Who are the "significant others" who serve as a support system for the client?

8. What health practices does the client regularly routinely engage in?

9. What does the client need to know to improve his or her self-care skills?

10. What barriers to self-care exist?

Each person comes equipped with a system of self-care already in place. Self-care may be culturally or scientifically based (Pender, 1987). For example, the patient may regularly read magazines, newspapers, and even health-oriented materials. At the other extreme, a patient may use folk medicine practices learned from family members. Thus, any self-care program must be compatible with the patient's life and his or her cultural, social, and environmental setting. For example, foods that are rich sources of protein can vary widely from culture to culture. Many approaches are available for dealing with stress. No single approach will fit all patients.

Next, it is helpful to understand the question of whether the concept of health (as opposed to illness) has any meaning for the patient. As Andrew Steptoe and Andrew Matthews of the Department of Psychology at St. George's Hospital Medical School at the University of London have suggested, certain behaviors that may affect a person's health may be undertaken or avoided for motives other than achieving health. For example, adults who brush their teeth every morning and several times every day, and who have done so since childhood, probably learned this behavior early in life, but for reasons not related to dental health. In the adult, the behavior is often triggered by the various stimuli associated with brushing the teeth: awakening, experiencing an undesirable taste, and so forth. As Steptoe and Matthews add, many behaviors that have implications for health, such as patterns of eating, exercising, or even smoking, are responses to social, environmental, and other influences and are to a great extent just habits (Steptoe & Mathews, 1984).

The next step is to get the patient's attention. Just as college lecturers learn they must get students' attention with the extremes of using costumes or dramatics (one chemistry professor sometimes resorts to a mild explosion to wake up students in the last row), nurses need to get a patient's full attention before they can focus on the subject at hand. The nurse can do this by telling a story or an anecdote or by asking the patient ahead of time to do some thinking about a particular subject and be prepared to talk about it at the next session.

Without the patient's attention, all the information in the world is of little use. A patient who is in a clinic setting, for example, will experience a wide range of physical and psychological barriers that compete with the nurse for attention (Rorden, 1987). A major barrier to overcome is the patient's lack of expectation that he or she will be learning anything. Unlike students in a classroom, who know they are in a learning setting, patients will not generally have the same level of expectation (Rorden, 1987). Unless they are prepared for the lesson, it is unlikely that they will automatically be ready to learn.

Patients are also generally in a highly stressful situation in a clinical setting. In such a case, patients generally will pay attention to teaching only if they perceive that the teaching will help reduce their level of stress. Attention span should also be considered, because even under the best of situations it is limited. Attention span varies not only with interest in the subject at hand but with time of day, room temperature, and fatigue, for example. At best, 45 min of concentrated attention is the most that can be expected (Rorden, 1987).

Next, it is helpful to clarify the objectives of the lesson. At the outset, it is important to let the patient know what to expect. One way is to clarify the behavior that is expected as a result of the lesson, for example, losing a certain number of pounds or learning how to take an antihypertensive drug. An "organizer" may be helpful at this stage. An organizer can be any of a number of materials that help clarify the lesson, such as a list of side effects caused by a drug and guidelines for taking the drug. Another type of organizer might be a list of foods, their calories per given quantity, and amounts allowed each day.

Then, the lesson can be presented, and feedback received. In order to underscore the lesson, it is helpful to give an example or an illustration to reinforce the material, such as the case of a patient with a similar health problem. Reinforcing learning is another important phase of any lesson. Reinforcing learning involves much more than just repeating several points; it means helping learners make the new knowledge, attitude, or health skill their own (Rorden, 1987). The best reinforcement is the practical, real-life application of the learned material to the learner's situation, with the guidance of the nurse.

A good learning situation should offer the patient an opportunity to try out new behaviors and to receive support and instruction from the staff (Rankin & Duffy, 1983). Unfortunately, what often happens is that the patient is instructed and shown the new skills, but remains in a dependent role. Then he or she is often discharged from the hospital without having had the chance to try out the

new behaviors. If a skill is being learned, it may be necessary for the patient come back for another demonstration, or it may be necessary to teach the patient and the patient's spouse a particular health skill. Learning will also be helped by involving as many of the learner's senses as possible. The reinforcement step is a chance to repeat the material or skill and to involve the patient emotionally and physically, and often intellectually, in his or her own care.

The final step is to summarize and evaluate the material in the lesson. Here, the teacher and student look back over the material and summarize what was learned. The major points in the lesson can be reemphasized, and both student and teacher can decide how well the objectives were met. Evaluating the lesson can be as simple and informal as briefly discussing the progress or as formal as a written statement (Rorden, 1987).

IMPROVING COMPLIANCE

Despite the best and most systematic approach to teaching, one of the most common complaints is that patients do not adhere to suggested lifestyle changes or are not motivated to learn new behaviors. Problems motivating patients or achieving compliance seem to be universal complaints of health care professionals.

How can patients be motivated to learn? An important place to start, according to Sally H. Rankin, assistant professor at the University of Southern California, Los Angeles, and Karen L. Duffy, program coordinator, staff education and development at Durham County General Hospital, Durham, NC, is to examine some of the characteristics of the adult learner. According to these two educators, many nurses teach patients and the patients' families in the ways the nurses were taught as children. The learners assume a passive role as the nurse lectures and demonstrates material to them, much as the nurse's teacher did in the grammar school or high school setting. Rankin and Duffy (1983) note the following:

> If the nurse tries to imagine herself as an adult student seated in a fifth-grade classroom, she will understand why the adult patient needs a different environment. She might imagine herself feeling anxious about what the teacher expects, concerned that the material may be repetitious and boring, and that the class schedule is rigid and her chair uncomfortable. She knows that she is not allowed to speak without permission. She feels that her past experience is not important and that she may have to learn things that are not relevant to her interests.

Characteristics of an adult learner. Adults seem to learn better when they can be self-directed in setting learning expectations, learn at their own pace, and have a voice in selecting learning resources (Redman, 1981). They also do better when they have an idea of the structure and process they will be working with, and when links can be made between organized knowledge and their own personal experiences, current knowledge, and new learning. With older adults, providing memory aids such as handouts combats the natural decline in short-term memory. With complex material, it often helps to provide categories and other structures to help them organize material. Finally, minimizing distracting and irrelevant information will be helpful (Redman, 1981).

When nurses consider their own positive learning experiences as adults, they are likely to recall an environment of comfort, physically and psychologically, where they were accepted students who felt valued and were encouraged to contribute their thoughts, ideas, and past experiences to the instructor and classmates. In addition, the subject matter was interesting and had a later application; that is, it could be used either on the job or in life in general. As Rankin and Duffy (1983) point out, with help, the nurses defined their own learning goals and evaluated the results of the learning activities, then had opportunities for role-playing or trying out new behaviors. They could ask questions without embarrassment and were encouraged to do so. Adult patients have similar needs as learners. They need physical and emotional comfort and a chance to actively participate in determining their own needs and goals, which motivates them to learn.

Educator Malcolm Knowles also outlines some guidelines about the adult learner that may be helpful in his book, *The Modern Practice of Adult Education.* As persons mature, their self-concept moves from dependency to self-direction. They see themselves as capable of making their own decisions, taking responsibility for the consequences, and managing their own lives. They gain life experiences that are an increasing resource for learning, and readiness to learn is increasingly oriented to their social roles. Their time perspective shifts so that they need to be able to immediately apply learning (rather than waiting to use the information at a later time), and their learning becomes problem centered rather than subject centered. In addition, adults view themselves as producers or doers and gain self-esteem from their contributions. They need to be perceived as in control of themselves, and they respond in an environment that is informal and friendly, where they are known by name and valued as individuals.

Adult learners are motivated to learn when they see there is an information gap between what they know and what they want to know (Rankin & Duffy, 1983). The information gained at the first meetings gives the nurse data about where patients stand with respect to the knowledge, attitudes, and skills they need for self-care.

Goals can be set and objectives devised. Goal setting is a method of contracting with patients to learn what they want to accomplish. It is also important to learn what the patient and the patient's family wish to accomplish. This will be influenced by their degrees of physical discomfort, denial, grieving, and dependency needs (Rankin & Duffy, 1983). We have only to think of the drastic example of Rosie, the middle-aged diabetic patient, to underscore this point. Nurse-educators should never try to force their own goals on a patient or the patient's family. Instead, the nurse should try to encourage whatever participation patients and their families can offer and consider ways to help them do so. Objectives are specific steps or statements related to a goal. For example, a goal may be to help a patient lose 25 lb by September. The objectives would be the menu, weekly clinic visits, and review of daily intake.

Goals and objectives tell patients clearly what the patients' role is and what is expected of them. Then they can organize their efforts toward accomplishing the goal. Sometimes setting a goal is the only intervention a nurse needs to direct the patient to a healthier lifestyle. Goals and objectives also help nurse-educators know their role. Both teacher and learner then have a method of knowing how to measure results.

Long- and short-term objectives should be outlined. That is, the short-term goals should fit into a specific long-term goal so that learning proceeds in a logical manner. Some educators use a goal-identification form. It states the overall or long-term goal, then lists the related short-term goals in very specific steps. For example, if the long-term goal for the patient is to take a brisk walk for 45 min four times a week, the patient can be given a form that spells out the short-term goals in clear detail. For example, the first short-term goal might be learning to take the pulse. Then, the next step would be to demonstrate two warm-up exercises to use before brisk walking begins, and so forth. Most forms like this also include an important section, a place where patients can write down the goals they have achieved.

Behavioral contracts. When new behaviors are determined that a client is willing to try, a verbal commitment to change is usually made. A written behavioral contract between nurse and client is a fairly recent development. With a behavioral contract, the person or client negotiates a realistic behavior change with another person or with himself or herself. Often patients find it is easier to follow through with a specific behavior if they have made a definite commitment to another person to do so or if they will be rewarded once they reach the goal. Goals must be achievable. For example, no healthful exercise program can enable a person to break a 4-min mile or to lose large amounts of weight within a short time.

A behavioral contract lists specific information: (a) the change to be made, (b) the way in which the change will be accomplished, (c) the person who is going to participate in the change, (d) the time frame in which the behavior will be accomplished, and (e) the consequences of meeting or not meeting the terms of the contract. Nurse-client contracts and self-contracts are the two most common types of behavioral contracts in use.

A nurse-client contract can be defined as any working agreement, continuously renegotiable, between nurse, client, and family (Pender, 1987). Such contracts specify the mutual objectives and responsibilities of each party to the contract. They are generally less formal than a typical legal contract and are not legally binding (unless fee negotiations are included). The object of the contract is to mutually involve the client and the nurse in a meaningful contract that helps the signers recognize the responsibility of the patient for the patient's own health and the caring, counseling, supportive role of the nurse. Such contracts also enable patients to actively participate in their own care by choosing realistic goals. The contract also makes clear who is responsible for what. Usually the client is responsible for carrying out certain behaviors, whereas the nurse is responsible for providing information, training, counseling, or specific reinforcements and rewards. The nurse is also responsible for providing helpful input and continuing feedback to the client about the client's performance and diligently managing the reinforcement and reward. Failing to do this destroys the trust and confidence the patient has in the nurse.

Contracts are usually devised after the client and nurse explore the client's health concerns and problems (family members may also participate in the discussion). Mutually agreeable goals are established, resources are determined, and a plan is devised to help the patient reach the goal. Responsibilities are negotiated, a mutually agreeable time frame is set, and mutual evaluation of progress toward accomplishing the goal is designated. Then, the contact is modified, renegotiated, or terminated.

The following characteristics are important in nurse-client contracts (Herje, 1980):

1. Goals should be realistic.

2. Behavior related to reaching goals should be measurable.

3. Goals should be stated in positive, rather than negative, terms.

4. The contract should contain a definite time frame for accomplishment.

5. The contract should be written and signed by both nurse and client, and a copy retained by each.

6. Behavior indicative of goal attainment should be rewardable.

7. The degree to which the goal is achieved must be able to be evaluated.

The contract also should provide incentives for behavioral change rather than relying merely on the patient's persistence and willpower. Rewards should be immediate as often as possible and should be reinforcing to the client. Although withholding rewards or reinforcement is usually considered fair by the client, penalties imposed for failure to perform can create resentment and hostility and may threaten the nurse-client relationship. Thus, subtle forms of punishment, such as promoting guilt or shame, or penalties should never be used with nurse-client contracts (Pender, 1987).

Family members can also be included in contracts. Family members provide an important source of encouragement, reinforcement, and reward and can be active participants through specific activities with the client. For example, a wife may agree to accompany her husband on brisk walks or entertain the children while he practices relaxation techniques to combat stress.

The contract itself must be periodically evaluated to see if it was effective. Did it accomplish the stated goals? If not, why? Can it be reorganized or renegotiated to be more successful? Sometimes a new contract is required.

Nurse-client contracts need not be limited to behavioral contracts. Some nurse-educators have had success with learning contracts. The learning contract, drawn between teacher (nurse) and student (patient), clearly states learning behaviors, the responsibilities of the teacher and the learner, and the methods of follow-up and evaluation. The contract is renegotiated as learning is accomplished and new goals are defined. If the patient changes his or her mind or finds that the goals can not be achieved, the objectives can be revised (Rankin & Duffy, 1983).

Self-contract. A self-contract is a commitment made by a person to himself or herself to perform specific behaviors for a previously specified reinforcement that is both attractive and motivating (DeRisi & Butz, 1975). With this approach, because the client is responsible for both making the commitment to behavior change and conveying the reward, immediate reinforcement is possible. Self-contracting does create a sense of independence and autonomy. With it, patients do not become overly dependent on a nurse to "police" their behavior.

Some patients are not good candidates for self-contracting. People who have low self-esteem or little perception of control over their health may not feel compelled to meet their own expectations and demands. Without the external expectations of others, there is little follow-through on specific activities to meet contract terms.

Control and learned helplessness. Control and learned helplessness are two powerful forces that may affect a patient's ability to comply with health suggestions. Control is a person's real or perceived ability to determine the outcome of an event. From early infancy, humans try to predict or control their environment and conditions of living (Pender, 1987). An infant's crying behavior is the earliest attempt to communicate with others to manipulate the environment and to attain human contact and proximity.

According to social learning theories, the concept of "locus of control" is used to explain the relationship between behavior and its outcome (Rotter, 1971). Unless people believe that their behavior directly affects their current state of health and future health, little motivation exists to engage in health-promoting and health-protecting behaviors. When behavior is perceived as causally linked to outcomes, perceptions of control are possible (Gatchel & Baum, 1983). When outcomes cannot be tied to behavior, it is much more difficult to believe that we are in control.

Perceptions of control of personal and family health are essential if patients are to assume the responsibility for self-care. Unfortunately, too often the health care setting produces just the opposite effect. This may be caused by condescending behavior, paternalistic attitudes, withholding of information, and the mystification of the health care experience (Pender, 1987). In such settings, patients remain in awe of the medical staff, and

view themselves almost like visitors to a "temple" that they must enter with reverence and deference to all who work there.

Research has shown that people tend to overestimate the degree of control they really have. Learned helplessness occurs when control is not available, or when persons cannot, under any condition, gain some sense of control over what happens to them. Repeated exposure to uncontrollable events conditions people to expect responses and outcomes to be noncontingent, and this produces learned helplessness. Patients can learn to be helpless, that is, learn that their attempts to succeed or control what happens to them will not be successful (Gatchel & Baum, 1983).

Studies of elderly people placed in nursing homes or hospitals have shown the effects of control and learned helplessness. When older persons are moved from their familiar settings into a new environment, they often lose their sense of control over their surroundings. If their new home is similar to their old one, it will be more predictable and as a result will seem more controllable to them. In addition, if steps are taken to give them a sense of control over their new environment, such as making them responsible for some aspect of it, or providing them with information about it, helplessness will be minimized and their health improved.

Learned helplessness suggests a number of links to health and illness. Prolonged or repeated exposure to settings or situations in which people have little or no control appears to be associated with reduced motivation, emotional disturbance, and cognitive impairment. When, however, helplessness is minimized by enhancing a person's sense of control, health outcomes appear to improve (Gatchel & Baum, 1983).

In his book *Helplessness: On Depression, Development, and Death* (W. H. Freeman and Company, 1975), M. E. Seligman gives an example of learned helplessness:

Major F. Harold Kushner, a medical army oficer who was captured and held as a prisoner of war for 5.5 years in South Vietnam. described a prisoner who became a victim of learned helplessness after careful manipulation by his captors. Major Kushner's story is one of the few cases on record in which a trained medical observer witnessed, from start to finish, death from helplessness.

Major Kushner was shot down in a helicopter in North Vietnam in November 1967. He spent the next 3 years in a hellish prisoner of war camp called First Camp. The camp's conditions were nearly beyond description. At any time, at least 11 men were crowded into a bamboo hut. The men slept on one crowded bamboo bed about 16 ft across. Their basic diet was three small cups of red, rotten, vermin-infested rice a day. Within the first year, the average prisoner lost 40–50% of his body weight and acquired running sores and atrophied muscles.

Major Kushner reported that there were two main killers of the prisoners: malnutrition and helplessness. When Kushner was first captured, he was asked to make antiwar statements. He said that he would rather die, and his captor responded, "Dying is easy; it is living that's hard."

Robert had been a captive and resident of First Camp for 2 years when Major Kushner was captured. Robert was a rugged and intelligent corporal from a crack marine unit and was described as austere, stoic, and nearly oblivious to pain and suffering. He was 24 years old and had been trained as a parachutist and a scuba diver. Like the rest of the prisoners, Robert weighed about 90 lb. The guards forced Robert to make long, shoeless treks daily with 90 lb of manioc root on his back. He never griped, but encouraged the other prisoners to grit their teeth and tighten their belts.

Despite malnutrition and a terrible skin disease, Robert remained in amazingly good physical and mental health. The cause of his relatively fine shape soon became clear to Major Kushner: Robert was convinced he would soon be released. The Viet Cong regularly released a few men who had cooperated with them and adopted the "correct" attitudes. They thus served as examples to the other prisoners. The prison camp commander had indicated that since Robert had cooperated, he was next in line for release in 6 months.

As expected, 6 months later, a high-ranking Viet Cong cadre appeared to give the prisoners a political course. It was understood that the outstanding pupil would be released after the course. Robert was chosen as the leader of the thought-reform group, and he made the required statements. The leader told Robert to expect release within the month.

The month came and went, and Robert began to sense a change in the guards' attitudes toward him. Finally it dawned on him that he had been duped. He had already served his captors' purpose and was not going to be released. He stopped working and showed signs of severe depression. He refused food and lay on his bed in a fetal position, sucking his thumb. His fellow prisoners tried to bring him around by hugging him, babying him, and giving him lots of attention. When this did not snap him out of his stupor, they tried striking him with their fists. He defecated and urinated in the bed. After a few weeks, Major Kushner knew that Robert was moribund. He was dusky and cyanotic.

One day, Robert sat up, asked Major Kushner to give a message to his family, then suddenly died. His death was typical of a number of deaths that Major Kushner witnessed. He was unable to perform an autopsy to learn the cause of death, because the Viet Cong allowed no surgical tools. However, Major Kushner suspected that learned helplessness had ultimately killed Robert. The apparent cause of death was electrolyte imbalance, but, given Robert's relatively good physical condition, psychologic rather than physiological factors seemed to have led to his death. When he gave up hope, when he believed that all his efforts had failed and would continue to fail, he died.

Learned helplessness has some implications for cardiac patients, too. Some may feel their disease is permanent and thus give up on diet or exercise plans or skip follow-up contacts.

How can learned helplessness be unlearned or reversed? Several studies in children have shown that it is possible to undo the effects of helplessness conditioning. In one study, fifth-grade children were given block design tasks similar to those associated with intelligence testing. Children were shown a picture of a design, given some multicolored blocks, and asked to form the design by using the blocks. The designs the children were asked to make could not be made with the blocks they were given. For children who blamed the problem on the environment, performance was worse than for children who took personal responsibility for their failure. Thus, when children believed that the failure to make the design was their own fault (e.g., that they had failed because they did not try hard enough), they continued to

work on other tasks.

This study suggested that it is possible to undo or reverse the effects of helplessness conditioning. If expectancies affect the response to failure, and a greater sense of personal responsibility leads to more persistent behavior, then training people to assume that their performance is determined largely by effort and ability could make them more resistant to the effects of lack of control. This approach can be applied to a patient whose efforts to lose weight or stop smoking or exercise more can be reinforced by seeing that his or her efforts do pay off.

Self-monitoring. In contrast to self-contracting, self-monitoring, the process of observing and recording one's own behavior, has formed a component of most self-control programs. It can be seen in one form in many diet programs, in which patients record the amounts and types of foods they consume each day. Some have hypothesized that self-monitoring can alter behavior. That is, persons can observe one of their behaviors, evaluate it, and then regulate it.

Reinforcement. Reinforcement can take a multitude of forms, from praise for a job well done or a self-administered treat for successful performance to a monetary penalty or loss of reward or aversive reinforcement or punishment for not carrying out a behavior. Behavior does tend to be regulated by its consequences, and people usually discard activities that are punished or unrewarded, while keeping those that are rewarded. It is easy to see why patients placed on preventive regimens could be the poorest compliers. Their daily health efforts go unrewarded, and the only motivating factor they may have is some (often vague) increased probability of avoiding an unpleasant consequence at some time in the distant future. Two good examples of this would be the stroke that attacks the hypertensive patient or the MI that results from high cholesterol levels.

Clients should be made aware of the importance of rewards or self-reinforcement in the health education process. They need to learn to reward their own efforts and achievements, because often the reward can not be supplied by others. Some nurses use a specific form that a patient can fill out ahead of time, listing the following: the goal or activity for the day, whether it was reached, and the reward for attaining the goal. The reward might be buying a new book or favorite perfume, visiting with a friend, or going to a movie. Patients should be discouraged from using food as a reward. Rewarding 30 min of jogging with a triple banana split is obviously self-defeating (Pender, 1987).

It is also important that clients learn to use internal as well as external self-reinforcement. Self-praise, complimenting oneself, and feeling good about oneself are forms of internal reinforcement. This also enables the client to be less dependent on tangible objects as rewards to learning. It is also helpful to get the family involved as sources of support for one another. For example, if the client achieves a goal, the reward might be a family trip to a local park or an overnight or weekend camping trip for the entire family. This helps create mutual support and a sense of healthy interdependence rather than crippling dependency (Pender, 1987). If home visits are not possible, the family should be encouraged to come to the clinic along with the patient.

Barriers to change. An earlier chapter focuses on the barriers to change that patients may erect. When the client does not seem to be making any progress, the nurse should explore possible barriers in the family setting, among support groups and friends, and in the patient's immediate environment. Nurses and clients should find time to talk about barriers that may arise and to deal with the barriers as the obstacles appear. Some patients may be reluctant to discuss the real reason they are not making any progress or may be unaware of some barriers. Establishing an open, empathetic atmos-

phere from the outset makes easier to communicate about obstacles to learning and progress.

A FEW FUNDAMENTALS

Certainly, helping patients change harmful habits and live longer and healthier lives can be a rewarding experience. For most nurses, teaching takes a little practice. If you have never taught a session or feel uncomfortable about doing so, there are some ways to start and to gain confidence in teaching. Barbara Redman suggests several steps you can take (1981). First, go along with another nurse who is known to be a good teacher and observe. Later ask questions about why each thing was done.

In the beginning, to build confidence, teach patients who have a common need to learn more about a subject in which you are an expert. Excellent teaching materials will help, too. Keep working. Become expert in a second, then a third area, and so forth. Write down the rationale for teaching and critique the approach.

No set rules can be laid down as absolute standards for effective teaching. However, educator Ruth Beckmann Murray (Murray & Zentner, 1985) has a few suggestions.

First, the nurse must assume that the best teaching device is the nurse. Patients can sense interest in them, and respond to the nurse's self-esteem and enthusiasm. it is important to know the subject area and to organize and present materials so that patients feel you know what to do. When the information needed is outside your expertise, ask an expert to take over to provide that part of the lesson or look for written materials or other information sources. For example, the nurse may want to explain how cardiac catheterization is performed. A nurse who specializes in that area can visit the patient or client to add information about that area. Many hospital and university medical center libraries have excellent videotapes and audiotapes that can be checked out for teaching sessions.

Here are a few more suggestions (Murray & Zentner, 1985):

1. Respect the client as more important than a procedure, a potential disease, or a research project.

2. Involve the client actively in the learning process.

3. If you ask the client to do something, give an explanation of why it is important. Be sure that what you ask is realistic.

4. Try to distinguish between lack of intelligence and misunderstanding caused by cultural, ethnic, or religious differences. Do not equate intelligence level with educational level. Don't allow racial bias to influence your opinion about another person's ability to learn.

5. Practice sensing the moment of learning. A good sense of timing is essential in teaching, based on your assessment of the learner's interest, knowledge, motivation, and values.

6. When you write out instructions, make sure they are legible.

7. Plan for interruptions.

8. Do not reinforce destructive thinking. For example, when the patient says, "My mother died of this disease," do not automatically reply, "Yes, it is a real killer. Two of my aunts died of it, too."

9. Keep notes during your teaching sessions and share these with other staff members or other teachers from other disciplines who may instruct the patient.

Finally, be realistic about teaching and learning. All nurses have good and bad days. Some days patients are more receptive, whereas other days they are distracted by problems at work or at home. Some days the teacher is elated and sometimes depressed by the results. Also, the nurse will not be able to reach all patients all the time, and sometimes patients disregard advice, skip sessions, or stop coming altogether. Finally, despite best efforts, some people are unwilling to attempt to change, or they may meet with such resistance from their families that they ultimately go back to the old lifestyle.

The final chapter turns to some of the national and local health programs that are having an impact on cardiovascular disease. It also briefly outlines some ways that nurses can help patients stick to programs aimed at changing harmful health behaviors.

EXAM QUESTIONS

CHAPTER 8
Questions 80–94

80. True or false: Many health care professionals are much better at presenting health care changes than at motivating patients to make such changes.

   a. True

   b. False

81. Which of the following is the best strategy for dealing with a cardiac patient who can not speak English?

   a. Ask another staff member to translate, or find a member of the patient's family who speaks English.

   b. Ask that the patient be transferred to another unit.

   c. Request that the patient be enrolled in an English class.

   d. Use only written materials for education.

82. Which of the following strategies can be used when a nurse first starts counseling a patient about lifestyle changes?

   a. Start with the area the nurse is most interested in.

   b. Start with the area of greatest concern to the patient.

   c. Skip all areas the patient is not concerned about.

   d. Try several different topics at the first meeting, to test the patient's interest level.

83. Which phase of the nurse-client relationship is the time when regular contacts between a nurse and client are gradually tapered off and ended?

   a. Transition

   b. Termination

   c. Action-reaction

   d. Renewal

84. True or false: Telephone contacts are often just as effective as face-to-face contacts.

   a. True

   b. False

85. One major barrier that will compete with a nurse's attempts to get the patient's attention is:

   a. The presence of family members

   b. The patient's lack of expectation that he or she will be learning anything

   c. The time of day

   d. The patient's age

86. Which of the following are characteristics of an adult learner?

   a. Adults are not bothered by distracting or irrelevant material.

   b. After age 25, people have less capacity to retain information.

   c. Adults do best with loosely structured materials.

d. Adults learn better when they have a chance to be self-directed.

87. True or false: A nurse-client contract is a continuously negotiable document.

a. True

b. False

88. Which of the following principles applies to a nurse-client contract?

a. The goals need only to be stated, not measurable.

b. The contract should be written and signed by both client and nurse.

c. The contract can contain a loose time frame, which is less threatening to the client.

d. The patient should write the contract without a witness.

89. True or false: Family members can be included in nurse-client contracts.

a. True

b. False

90. Which of the following persons might **not** be a good candidate for a self-contract?

a. An independent, self-sufficient person

b. A patient who is not fluent in English

c. An overweight male

d. A person with low self-esteem

91. True or false: Research has shown that people tend to overestimate the degree of control they have.

a. True

b. False

92. How does self-monitoring differ from self-contracting?

a. Self-monitoring involves observing and recording one's own behavior and does not involve a "contract."

b. Self-monitoring must be done in a group setting.

c. Self-monitoring is reserved for a few, select patients, whereas self-contracting is applicable to anyone.

d. Self-monitoring is aimed at younger and healthier patients, whereas self-contracting is limited to older adults.

93. Which of the following strategies will help a nurse who is not experienced in teaching?

a. Reading as many education textbooks as possible

b. At first, teaching patients who have a common need to learn about a subject the nurse is expert in

c. Teaching only one patient at a time

d. Ask the physician to educate the patient

94. True or false: Changes in daily health habits are affected more by the patient's environment than by visits to health care professionals.

a. True

b. False

CHAPTER 9

PREVENTING CARDIOVASCULAR DISEASE

CHAPTER OBJECTIVE

After studying this chapter, the reader will be able to describe some methods for helping patients permanently change behaviors that place them at high risk for CHD.

LEARNING OBJECTIVES

After studying this chapter, the reader should be able to

1. List at least two characteristics that indicate a patient is willing to change his or her behavior.

2. Give three strategies that can be used to help promote cardiovascular health.

INTRODUCTION

Can health care professionals really make a difference in the battle against heart disease? The answer from studies thus far is a resounding yes. Deaths from CHD and stroke in the United States fell by 30% and 31.5%, respectively, in the decade between 1979 and 1989, according to the AHA (1992). Better health education and earlier intervention to help patients recognize and change risk factors have made a difference, as seen in the 20% decrease in all forms of heart disease between 1976 and 1986 (AHA, 1988).

Despite these successes, much remains to be done, because atherosclerosis, a largely preventable progressive disease, is still so widespread in industrialized nations. It is estimated that about 1 million Americans die of cardiovascular disease annually (NHLBI, 1990). In addition, among adults, 38% of African-American men and 39% of African-American women have high blood pressure (AHA, 1988). The cost of treating cardiovascular diseases in 1989 was expected to be about $88.2 billion, according to the AHA; this included $56.3 billion in hospital and nursing home care and $12.5 billion in physician and nursing services, with $4.4 billion in medication costs.

Because evidence of atherosclerosis can be detected early in life, the effort to counteract the elements that can be changed, diet, exercise, and stress, must begin at an early age. The emphasis today is on primary prevention rather than on treatment once the disease process is well under way.

The concept of primary prevention was outlined more than 20 years ago. Primary prevention means intervening to change risks before disease or illness occurs and is designed to prevent or at least delay the onset of illness. Such a health-promotion strategy is often nonspecific and geared toward raising the general level of health and well-being of an individual, family, or community. An example of this would be teaching elementary school children about their bodies through a "Know Your Body" curriculum. On the community level, the most familiar example would be a vaccination program. By these programs, diseases such as small-pox have been virtually eliminated from the planet. Other examples might be campaigns to get motorcycle riders to wear helmets and purification of water supplies.

Programs to educate the general public about heart disease have been extremely successful at all levels. This final chapter looks at a few programs aimed at intervening against heart disease and reviews some of the ways nurses can help patients develop health strategies and adhere successfully to health-promoting programs.

PREVENTION: A NATIONWIDE EFFORT

The battle against heart disease has been waged at all levels in the United States and abroad. Local, state, and national efforts to educate Americans about the hazards of an overly rich diet, too little exercise, cigarette smoking, and high levels of stress have shown some promising results. There has been a downturn in the total annual number of deaths attributable to atherosclerosis since 1984 (AHA, 1987). Large-scale projects to detect and change the risk of CHD, such as the ongoing Framingham study, have underscored this, even while educating participants about the benefits of changing their lives to prevent heart disease.

Statewide programs such as the Heart Healthy Vermonter Program or Maryland's Healthy People Program have made an impact by helping educate state residents about heart disease. Locally, nearly every hospital or medical center of any size offers low-cost or free courses on atherosclerosis and weight reduction, and many offer exercise classes as well. Most also offer screening for diabetes and hypertension.

THREE PROGRAMS THAT HAVE MADE A DIFFERENCE

In Vermont, Maryland, and California, programs to help reduce heart disease risk factors have produced some promising results. The programs in Maryland and Vermont had small budgets and were designed to make use of local programs already in place.

The Heart Healthy Vermonter Program. Heart disease is the leading cause of morbidity and morality among Vermont residents, just as it is throughout America (Thompson, Hamrell, & Coffin, 1987). In 1984, for example, 37% of all deaths in Vermont were attributed to heart disease, and 46% were attributed to all classes of cardiovascular disease. When a telephone poll was taken in 1982 of 1,600 residents of Vermont, it was learned that 39% were overweight, 33% smoked cigarettes regularly, 70% got little or no exercise, 70% used whole milk, and 83% used hard margarine or butter (Novick et al., 1985).

The Heart Healthy Vermonter program was designed to intervene at the community level to prevent or delay cardiovascular disease by using three major components: community organization and education, professional education, and media development. The overall goal of the Heart Healthy Vermonter Program was to prevent premature heart attacks and deaths among Vermonters under the age of 65. The early emphasis was on primary prevention, targeted at the general public rather than at detecting and treating high-risk individuals.

The Vermont program revolved around providing information about healthy behaviors, designing training programs to help patients adopt such behaviors, and creating an environment that makes such changes easier. Five types of programs were offered at the community level. The first, "Heart Healthy Vermonter Eating Style," was a 6-week course that offered information about nutrition and heart disease, including instructions on menu planning, food preparation, recipe adaptation, and eating out. Next, the program adapted the AHA's healthy restaurant menu program. A volunteer registered dietitian consulted with each cooperating restaurant and monitored its compliance. At least 46 major restaurants in the state were participating by 1987 (Thompson et al., 1987).

The third program involved a wide-scale hypertension screening program in a number of communities. Screening was offered at many local points, including hospitals. Each person who participated in screening also received education, referral, and follow-up by a health care professional. More than 20,000 people have been screened for hypertension in 5 years.

Programs for screening, referral, and treatment of hyperlipidemia had been in place for years, yet program officials found a great deal of confusion and different modes of treating elevated serum cholesterol levels among health care professionals. There was even more disagreement about when therapy, especially with diet, should be begun. To counteract this, an annual symposium was offered for health professionals to increase and upgrade their knowledge about risk factors and heart diseases and to suggest up-to-date strategies for intervention.

A "Quit Smoking and Win" contest, with a drawing for prizes for those who quit smoking for at least a month, was featured. All prizes were donated by local businesses, and the grand prize winner received a trip for two to Hawaii. Each community agency also offered fitness events that drew attention to the importance of exercise for healthier hearts. In one community, the special event was "Surf/Sail for Heart Health," where residents were asked to make pledges to support a sailboarder who attempted to sail the length of Lake Champlain. This program helped raise money to support the project.

Finally, an effort was made to use the media to create awareness of heart disease and to inform and persuade Vermonters to adopt healthier lifestyles. Television was seen as a particularly important medium, and several public service announcements and campaigns were begun on cable and major television channels. One of the most popular programs was a program where local chefs from well-known restaurants demonstrated ways to prepare heart-healthy meals. Other promotional activities included a quarterly newsletter, bumper stickers, T-shirts, library displays, pamphlets and fliers, and days when local radio stations devoted all public service time to one risk factor for heart disease.

The programs that have generated the most interest and thus have been most successful in Vermont have been "environmental" activities. These activities have been defined as those that improve a person's environment, such as establishing designated smoking areas and labeling low-fat foods in restaurant menus. The second most successful type involved community-wide participation, including events promoted on a community-wide basis, such as fitness activities and health fairs. Activities aimed at individuals that attempted to change personal behaviors have been much more sparsely attended but have been continued because of indications that as people become more aware of heart health, they become more interested in making health care changes on their own.

The Healthy People Program in Maryland. The Healthy People Program targeted three major areas for change in several Maryland communities: cigarette smoking, obesity, and stress. In August 1981, the program was begun with a relatively low budget, $130,000–$175,000 annually for 4 years. The target audience was adult males, who were at greatest risk of heart disease, and a secondary risk group, pre-high school students, was targeted for an antismoking campaign. The project used pre-

and posttests, annual fitness tests, and mid-year and 1-year follow-up surveys for smoking and weight control programs.

In 1984, a task force conducted a smoking cessation program in Baltimore, a city of 2.2 million. This campaign was conducted to persuade smokers to make a pledge to quit smoking for 2 weeks as a start to quitting for life. More than 200,000 brochures with tear-off pledge cards were printed and distributed at work sites, retail stores, post offices, and libraries. Radio and television stations aired spots to persuade smokers to send in pledge cards and to call the Cancer Information Service for more information. Each person who called or sent in a pledge card received the "Quit for Good" stop-smoking pamphlets from the National Cancer Institute. Another quit-smoking program, "Quit and Win," offered a prize drawing for smokers who sent in a pledge card. These two programs led to a quit rate of between 6% and 13% (Buxton & Pfeffer, 1987). The researchers also found that the most successful programs were those that were begun at work sites.

To try to reach teenagers before they started smoking, the American Lung Association and the Maryland Project developed a peer-resistance smoking prevention program for sixth-grade students, "Smoking Deserves a Smart Answer." A program aimed at seventh graders, called Project SMART, was designed to help prevent use of tobacco, alcohol, and marijuana. A combination of the sixth- and seventh-grade programs aimed to reduce the smoking onset rate by 80%.

The second area targeted was excess weight. First, the researchers studied existing programs in 10 communities and learned that half of the participants of weight control groups regularly dropped out. One fourth of those entering the program, including the dropouts, lost weight, and half of those who lost weight maintained the loss (an average of 10 lb) for at least 6 months.

In an attempt to counteract these dropout rates, a weight-loss competition and incentive program, "Lose Weight and Win," was conducted. In this program, people who were overweight were invited to deposit $5 and to form a team of 10–14 people, who would weigh in every week for 10 weeks. Each week, the percentage of weight lost by each team was posted on a large board. The team that lost the highest percentage of its weight-loss goal at the end of the program was awarded the deposits.

The weight-loss program was the most successful portion of the statewide program. Twenty-one percent and 27% of the participants in the 1984 and 1985 programs, respectively, lost at least 10 lb during the 10 weeks. The average weight loss was approximately 6 lb in both programs.

A program to improve cardiovascular fitness and upper body strength was developed during 1982 and 1983 at the request of the Maryland Army National Guard. This program used incentives such as T-shirts and recognition, competition among companies and individuals, training at monthly drills, and annual fitness scores that could eventually influence promotions to improve the exercise levels of National Guard members. After 2.5 years, the National Guard assumed independent operation of the program. Between 1984 and 1986, the percentage of members passing the Army Readiness Test increased by 37%.

A brisk walking program was designed for the general public. This featured 12 walks in downtown Baltimore. About 90% of participants were women, and about 10% to 20% completed 9 of 12 walks.

Finally, a group stress-reduction program was developed. This program was designed to introduce stress-reduction strategies into organizations where risk-behavior changes might in turn be started. After a 1-year effort, most staff members decided that stress reduction was the lowest priority area, and members were transferred into stop-smoking programs. A booklet containing strategies for reducing stress was produced and distributed.

The Stanford Heart Disease Prevention Program. In the mid-1970s, three relatively isolated northern California towns of 12,000–15,000 people were studied in an attempt to reduce cardiovascular risk by reducing cigarette smoking, blood cholesterol levels, and elevated blood pressure (Maccoby, Farquhar, & Wood, 1977). The overall goal was to develop and evaluate methods to "influence the adult population at large to change their living habits in ways that would reduce their risk of premature heart attack and stroke" (Breslow, 1978).

In two communities, an intense media campaign against heart disease was used for more than 2 years, including face-to-face counseling about heart disease risk. The third community acted as a control. In the first two communities, individuals 35–59 years old who had increased risk of heart disease received face-to-face counseling. These at-risk individuals were detected through a baseline survey that included a behavioral interview and a medical examination. The survey included relevant information about attitudes and knowledge of risk-related behavior related to diet, weight, smoking, and exercise.

In 1972, a mass-media campaign was started in the two noncontrol communities to teach specific behavioral skills as well as to disseminate information and to affect attitudes about risk-related behaviors. The campaign involved television and radio "spots," hour-long programs, weekly newspaper columns, newspaper advertisements, billboards, posters, and printed materials that were mailed directly to residents. In one community, a random sample of those in the top quartile (top 25%) of risk were recruited for intensive face-to-face instruction.

Two subsequent annual surveys showed favor-

able changes in the physical variables that made up the risk and in specific knowledge and behavior. After 2 years, the degree of health knowledge was evaluated in all three communities. In the control community, knowledge had improved by 6%. In contrast, in the two communities where the campaign had been conducted, knowledge improved by 26–41%, and among those who had had intensive face-to-face counseling, it improved 54% (Breslow, 1978).

During the 2 years of the study, consumption of saturated fats and cholesterol declined 20–40% in the campaign communities, which was significantly greater than in the control community. This decrease was particularly high among high-risk men who had undergone intense instruction. Mean changes in serum cholesterol were highly correlated with the self-reported changes in dietary behavior.

Cigarette smoking also declined to a greater extent among the campaign towns than in the control community: In the two campaign communities, smoking declined 7–24%, but in the control community, smoking declined only 2.4%.

In the control community, the risk for CHD actually **increased** more than 5% during the 2 years of the study. In contrast, the risk in campaign communities declined 15–20% among all participants. The decline in risk was greatest in the groups that had had intense instruction about risk. Thus, the Stanford study showed that intervention by health care professionals, using educational media, could make a startling difference in the risk for CHD.

These three programs are examples of successful interventions made at the state and community levels. See *Table 17*, for hints for improving health promotion strategies. This is fine on a large scale, but how can individual nurses work on a one-to-one basis help patients change behaviors that place the patients at risk of heart disease?

HELPING PATIENTS CHANGE

Health care professionals are far more successful at prescribing healthy behavior changes than at motivating patients to adopt more healthful living habits (Zifferblatt, 1983). Patients and nurses alike know what healthful habits are because information about health abounds. The much more difficult part is getting patients to change and to adopt new behaviors.

Changes in daily habits are largely affected by the people and events that surround a patient each day, not by the time spent in a health education lecture once a month. Change also takes a long time. It may take years of repeated effort and often frustration until the right combination of motivating factors occurs (Zifferblatt, 1983). Most adults do think about the benefits of changing their health habits and often consider making changes. Sometimes they make an attempt to change, persist for a time, then go back to the old habits. Certainly the high dropout rate from most weight-loss programs reflects this.

Personal change is, after all, difficult for anyone. It is almost always much easier to keep old, familiar, comfortable lifelong habits than to substitute a new activity, even when the change is important. Change is most likely to occur when (a) old habits produce clearly adverse consequences, and (b) the potential benefits of new health habits markedly outweigh the benefits of keeping old health habits (Zifferblatt, 1983). Change also brings on anxiety and insecurity and creates the

---

Table 17

Hints for Improving Your Health Promotion Strategies

1. Increase the amount of patient teaching to include topics other than the reason for admission. Ask coworkers to cover your other patients while you teach. Then, be willing to return the favor. Ask supervisory personnel for additional staff coverage so that you can do patient teaching.

2. Keep health information readily available on your nursing unit. Pamphlets that address cigarette smoking, high blood pressure, arthritis, and cancer may be obtained from your local American Heart Association, American Cancer Society, and Arthritis Foundation.

3. Provide a lifestyle assessment tool (such as Health Risk or Health Hazard Appraisal) for all patients.

4. Remember that patients make their own decisions about health practices. Provide information and listen, but respect their choices.

5. Be a good role model. Assess your own lifestyle and work on modifications to make yourself healthier, but do not be overzealous in telling patients how far you run each day or how you stopped smoking.

6. Do not be afraid to talk about lifestyle with your patients. Remember that many are in the hospital because of lifestyle-induced diseases. Use the information on the data base for long-term as well as short-term planning.

7. Continue to give high-quality, skilled care. Your skilled care may be the reason your patients become well enough to assess their future health practices.

Source: Flynn, J. B., & Giffin, P. A. (1984). *Nursing Clinics of North America, 19,* 239-250.

real risk and threat of failure.

Furthermore, people have different motives for engaging in the same behaviors (Redman, 1981). In addition, it is not unusual for a person to have multiple motivating factors for a single behavior. How can nurses recognize patients who are most likely to successfully change their behavior? Barbara Redman has pinpointed four characteristics that indicate a person who is most likely to change behavior (Redman, 1981). According to her, behavioral change is most likely to occur when persons:

1. Are intrinsically motivated, or want to feel competent in dealing with their environment.

2. Are mastering the tasks of their developmental stage and the tasks of adapting to their illness.

3. Have beliefs about health that agree with those of the caregiver and have a fairly high knowledge level in the health beliefs system.

4. Have environments that can be supportive in helping them attain and maintain the new behavior, thus creating ongoing rewards for that behavior.

Health habits also are formed by environmental variables–cultural, historical, economic, and social—as well as for hedonistic, or pleasurable, reasons. It may be impossible to establish the origin of health-related behavior on a scientific basis, because each time it seems that one factor is isolated, it often turns out to be related to another (Zifferblatt, 1983).

The following are five brief guidelines (Zifferblatt, 1983) to keep in mind when trying to help patients change their behaviors:

1. Patients must accept responsibility for changing their daily health habits. At the beginning, the nurse must have a frank and direct discussions with patients to clarify that the patients, and not the nurse, bear primary responsibility for changing daily health habits. It is helpful to stress that changing habits requires a direct, daily effort for at least 6 months and that initial efforts may be ineffective and frustrating. Sometimes, of course, once patients are aware that changes, such as stopping smoking or losing 45 lb, are difficult, they may decide not to go through with the program. When this happens, the door should be left open for counseling at any future date. It is impossible to predict when patients are ready to change, and an "open door" policy is the best.

2. Health care professionals must have data from patients to plan a strategy to help change behavior. The information-gathering process, starting with the family and personal histories, and specific tests are discussed in several chapters in this course. In addition, it is often helpful to have the patient keep a daily log or diary that correlates places, times, and even people with specific health behaviors. In this way, patients become involved in working on the solution to their own problems, and their active participation increases the likelihood that they will comply or follow through on specifically suggested courses of action. If, on the other hand, they do not want to invest the time or effort in a daily diary, it is easy to assume that they will not be willing to follow through on recommended behavior changes or new behaviors. If patients are willing to go to the trouble to keep a daily diary, the data they collect should be used in some way in the program.

3. A gradual approach to change is best. As cardiologist Steven Zifferblatt (1983) says, "A graduated approach is the treatment of choice when the patient is willing, because it is easier to build long-lasting motivation on probable success than on probable failure." The patient's past performance should guide the next step in treatment, and the increments toward the treatment goal can never be too small. In contrast, a very enthusiastic patient may try to do too

much too quickly, and fail, rather than taking a measured, stepwise approach and succeeding.

4. Change must last for at least 6 months before it can be considered a reality. The 6-month mark may be the first serious hurdle the patient faces. Talking about hurdles and discussing strategies of facing and overcoming them as they arise can be reassuring and can prevent the disappointments that may occur when a goal is not met or is almost met. There is no easy or pat formula for behavior change, or for achieving permanent behavior changes, and patients need to be taught that the key is commitment and persistence, not an easy "fix."

5. Permanent change often means that patients will have to restructure the world they live in. Patients may need to build social, emotional, and physical support systems to reinforce and protect desired behavioral changes. It is not unusual for patients to be highly anxious when dealing with the threat of, or the actual loss of, a significant part of their health. In such a case, patients can be easily overwhelmed and may give up on education. They can be helped with memory support, easy and concrete tasks, clear directions, and instructor feedback about what and how they are doing. It is a good idea to encourage patients to keep in contact by phone and with regular visits, whether or not they are having problems with their program of change. A supportive environment allows easy access to information, including availability to answer questions, and easy access to medical personnel in getting appointments. You may recall the earlier example of noncompliance at a hypertension clinic; one of the major objections of the participants was that they often had to wait 45 min before they could speak to a physician.

6. Honesty and openness are essential to success. They develop at the first meetings with patients, where a climate of trust and acceptance is created. For patients who are learning new treatment regimens, consciously assess compliance at every follow-up visit. For example, the nurse can ask, "What medicines are you taking?" "How often?" "Do you have any problems taking them every day?"

Also, do not avoid eliciting negative feedback. Consider asking about any side effects from their new regimen, dissatisfaction with treatment, concerns they feel have not been dealt with, and any questions. The more specific the questions are, the more likely you will be able to elicit negative feedback. It is often a good idea to reserve detailed questions for times when things are not going well or when you suspect patients are not taking their medication.

Finally, remember that any successful program takes time. Each patient progresses at a different speed and brings different degrees of knowledge and experience and levels of health to the project. Setting realistic goals and having realistic expectations help both patients and nurses increase the probability of success.

EXAM QUESTIONS

CHAPTER 9
Questions 95–100

95. Under what circumstances will behavioral change most likely occur?

    a. The patient's beliefs about health agree with the caregiver's beliefs.

    b. The patient knows the possible adverse outcome of his or her behavior.

    c. The patient seems ready to learn.

    d. The patient is an elderly adult.

96. True or false: It is not necessary for patients to accept responsibility for changing their daily health habits.

    a. True

    b. False

97. How can keeping a daily log or diary help change behavior?

    a. It keeps a patient's mind off the changes, thus reducing stress.

    b. It is a way for the nurse to check up on the patient's progress.

    c. The patient cannot share the information with family members and thus does not get immediate reinforcement for the unwanted behavior.

    d. The patient becomes involved in working on the solution to his or her problems.

98. True or false: A rapid change in health habits is best because it helps the patient reach his or her goals more rapidly.

    a. True

    b. False

99. For a behavioral or lifestyle change to be considered a reality, it should last for how long?

    a. 6 weeks

    b. 3 months

    c. 6 months

    d. 1 year

100. Which of the following statements about a permanent change in lifestyle is correct?

    a. It often means patients will have to restructure their environment.

    b. It is nearly impossible to attain.

    c. It must be made before age 50.

    d. It must include an ongoing education program.

APPENDIX

GENERAL DIET GUIDELINES

1. Avoid being overweight; consume only as many calories as you expend. If overweight, decrease calories and increase expenditure (e.g., exercise more).

2. Increase your consumption of fruits, vegetables, and whole grains (complex carbohydrates and "naturally occurring" sugars) from the present 28% of calories in the average diet to about half (48%) of your caloric intake.

3. Decrease your consumption of refined and other processed sugars and foods high in such sugar by almost half (about 45%) to account for only about 10% of your total calories.

4. Decrease your consumption of foods high in total fat from 42% of calories to 30% of calories.

5. Specifically reduce saturated* fat in your diet (from the present 16–10%), and partially replace this with polyunsaturated and monounsaturated fat to account for the remaining 20% of fat intake, by reducing intake of animal fat from meats and high-fat dairy products. Eat more fish and poultry, and select lean meats low in fat (e.g., trimmed ground round in place of hamburger). Low-fat and nonfat milk be substituted for whole milk except in those infants whose diet is almost entirely milk.

6. Reduce cholesterol to about 300 mg/day. (The major dietary sources of cholesterol are egg yolks, meats, whole milk, and high-fat dairy products.)

7. Decrease your consumption of salt and foods high in salt content from the present 6–18 g/day to about 5 g/day.

Saturated and unsaturated refer to the chemical structure of the fatty acid. A saturated fat has no double bonds, a monounsaturated fat has one double bond, and a polyunsaturated fat has two or more double bonds.

Source: The information in this appendix can be found in American Heart Association. (1986). The American Heart Association Heart Book. Dallas, TX: Author.

High-Sodium Foods to Avoid or Use Sparingly

Meats: Salted or smoked meats, bacon, bologna, corned beef, ham, luncheon meats, sausage, and salt pork.

Fish: Salted or smoked fish, anchovies, sardines, dried cod, and herring.

Flavorings: Commercial bouillon; catsup; chili sauce; celery, onion, or garlic salts; meat extracts, sauces, or tenderizers, unless low-sodium dietetic; prepared mustard; relishes; salt substitutes; cooking wine.

Cheeses: Processed cheese, cheese spreads, Roquefort, Camembert, and other strong cheeses.

Vegetables: Pickles, sauerkraut, and any other vegetables salted or packed in brine.

Miscellaneous: Peanut butter, unless low-sodium dietetic; breads or crackers with salt topping; potato chips; popcorn; pretzels; salted nuts; and olives.

Sodium: Some Points to Remember

1. Milk, meats, fish, cheese, and eggs are quite high in sodium.

2. Vegetables, breads, and cereals have moderate amounts of sodium. There is considerable variation among the different vegetables.

3. Fruits and fats are low in sodium or have only trace amounts.

4. Highly salted snack foods should be avoided.

5. Halve the amount of salt, soy sauce, and monosodium glutamate used in cooking and at the table.

6. Do not add salt to foods already salted in freezing and canning.

7. Try different flavorings instead of salt.

8. Do not use a salt substitute unless a physician has recommended it.

9. When eating out or buying prepared canned or frozen foods, try to avoid those with an unlisted salt content.

Hints on Lowering Intake of Cholesterol and Saturated Fats

1. Foods of plant origin do not contain cholesterol, and, except for coconut and palm oils, saturated fats are not high in plants. (However, vegetable oils may be artificially saturated or "hardened" by hydrogenation.) Use natural unprocessed foods of plant origin liberally.

2. Foods of animal origin, eggs, meats, and dairy products, are generally high in cholesterol and saturated fats. Eggs and organ meats are the highest in cholesterol. Shrimp is high in cholesterol, but low in fat. Use animal products sparingly, and for those you use, discard the high-fat, high-cholesterol parts, such as with eggs.

   a. Discard egg yolks.

   b. Do not eat organ meats (liver, kidney, brain, heart).

   c. Buy only the leanest meats (round steak instead of hamburger), and trim away all visible fat. Three ounces of lean red meat (cooked weight or 4 oz uncooked) three times per week is your allotment if you are at high risk.

   d. Protein-rich foods are usually taken at least twice per day. For your remaining 11 servings, instead of meat choose the following substitutes: Use skinned poultry (the skin is high in cholesterol and fat), preferably chicken or turkey white meat. (Avoid duck and goose; they are too fatty.) Use white fish. (But avoid lobster and shrimp, and go easy on other shellfish.) Use low-fat, uncreamed cottage cheese and, more cautiously, processed low-fat, low-cholesterol cheeses, such as Lite-Line. Even those at high risk may use Parmesan, mozzarella (part skim), and ricotta (part skim) in moderation. Use no more than 2 oz per week of cheddar or Swiss and other similar cheeses. Use vegetable proteins such as beans, peas, and "fake meats."

3. Totally exclude butter and lard. Avoid palm and coconut oil products (e.g., whipped toppings, some nondairy creamers). Use liquid oils and margarines high in polyunsaturates (especially those that come in tubs). When a recipe requires a hardened oil, use the least saturated forms (e.g., corn oil stick margarine). Stay away from hydrogenated margarines and shortening. Avoid prepared deep-fried foods and fried snack foods.

4. Use skim milk, not whole milk, or 2% milk. Do not use cream.

5. Avoid ice cream, cream pies, commercial cakes, and other sweets made with eggs and fat.

Cholesterol Content of Edible Single Portions of Selected Foods

Food	Cholesterol (mg)
Brains, raw	572.0
Egg yolks, fresh	429.0
Chicken livers, cooked	233.0
Kidneys, cooked	229.0
Egg, whole, fresh	157.0
Sweetbreads (thymus), cooked	133.0
Liver, beef and pork, cooked	125.0
Caviar or roe	103.0
Ladyfingers	101.0
Heart, beef, cooked	78.0
Butter	72.0
Sponge cake	71.0
Pie, lemon chiffon	48.0
Cheese souffle	48.0
Shrimp, boiled	43.0
Popovers	42.0
Sardines, canned in oil	40.0
Heavy whipping cream	38.0
Cream cheese	32.0
Custard, baked	30.0
Turkey, cooked	30.0
Crab, canned	29.0
Cheese, Swiss	29.0
Lamb or veal, cooked	28.0
Cheese, cheddar	28.0
Beef, cooked	27.0
Mackerel, canned	27.0
Chicken, dark meat, cooked	26.0
Cheese, brick	26.0
Pork, cooked	25.0
Cheese, blue	25.0
Brownies, with nuts	24.0
Lobster, cooked	24.0
Chicken, white meat, cooked	23.0
Pancakes	21.0
Mayonnaise	20.0
Corn bread	20.0
Sour cream	19.0
Tuna, in oil, drained	19.0
Frankfurter, raw	19.0
Clams, canned	18.0
Oysters, cod, flounder, halibut	14.0
Ice cream	14.0
Margarine (2/3 animal fat)	14.0

Chocolate cake with icing	13.0
Cream, half and half	13.0
Scallops or salmon, raw	10.0
Ice milk	6.0
Milk, whole	4.0
Milk, 2%; low-fat cottage cheese	3.0
Yogurt, low-fat, plain	2.0
Milk, skim	0.6

When a recipe calls for   Use

Sour cream Low-fat cottage cheese blended until smooth, or cottage cheese plus low-fat yogurt for flavor, or ricotta cheese made from partially skimmed milk (thinned with yogurt or buttermilk, if desired).

One can of chilled, evaporated skim milk whipped with 1 teaspoon of lemon juice. Low-fat buttermilk or low-fat yogurt.

Chocolate Cocoa blended with polyunsaturated oil or margarine (one 1-oz. square of chocolate = 3 tablespoons of cocoa + 1 tablespoon polyunsaturated oil or margarine).

Butter Polyunsaturated margarine or oil. One tablespoon butter = 1 tablespoon margarine.

Eggs Use commercially produced cholesterol-free egg substitutes according to package directions. Or use 1 egg white plus 3 teaspoons of polyunsaturated oil.

Milk Use 1 cup skim or nonfat dry milk plus 2 tablespoons of polyunsaturated oil as a substitute for 1 cup of whole milk.

Buttermilk One cup lukewarm nonfat milk plus 1 tablespoon of lemon juice = 1 cup buttermilk. Let the mixture stand for 5 min and beat briskly.

Cornstarch Use 1 tablespoon flour for $1^1/_2$ teaspoons cornstarch or 1 tablespoon arrowroot for 1 tablespoon cornstarch.

Cream cheese Blend 4 tablespoons of margarine with 1 cup dry low-fat cottage cheese. Add salt to taste and a small amount of skim milk if needed in blending mixture. Vegetables such as chopped chives or pimiento and herbs and seasonings can be added for variety.

BIBLIOGRAPHY

Adams, M. M. (1988, April). The forgotten victims of a medical crisis, *RN 1988,* pp. 30-39.

Aho, W. R. (1977). Relationships of wives' preventive health orientation to the beliefs about heart disease in husbands. *Public Health Reports, 92,* 65-71.

American Heart Association. (1981). *1981 heart facts.* Dallas: Author.

American Heart Association. (1986). *The American Heart Association heart book.* Dallas: Author.

American Heart Association. (1987). *1987 heart facts.* Dallas: Author.

American Heart Association. (1988). *1988 heart facts.* Dallas: Author.

American Heart Association. (1990). *National cholesterol education for nurses teaching materials.* Dallas: Author.

American Heart Association. (1992). *1992 heart and stroke facts,* Dallas: Author.

American Heart Association. (1992). Guidelines for cardiopulmonary resuscitation and emergency cardiac care. *Journal of the American Medical Association, 268* (16).

Anitschkow, N. (1933). Experimental arteriosclerosis in animals. In E. V. Cowdry (Ed.), *Arteriosclerosis* (pp. 271-322). New York: Macmillan.

Armstrong, M. L. (1976). Connective tissue in regression. *Arteriosclerosis Reviews, 1,* 147-168.

Aronow, W. S. (1971). Heart rate and carbon monoxide level after smoking high-, low-, and non-nicotine cigarettes: A study in male patients with angina pectoris. *Annals of Internal Medicine, 74,* 697-702.

Aronow, W. S. (1980). Effect of non-nicotine cigarettes and carbon monoxide on angina. *Circulation, 61,* 262-265.

Aronow, W. S., & Kaplan, N. M. (1983). Smoking. In N. M. Kaplan & J. Stamler (Eds.), *Prevention of coronary heart disease: Practical management of the risk factors.* Philadelphia: Saunders.

Ascah, K. J. (1988). Doppler echocardiography. In D. D. Miller, R. J. Burns, & J. B. Gill (Eds.), *Clinical cardiac imaging.* New York: McGraw-Hill.

Barger, A. C., Beewkes, R. III, Lainey, L. L., et al. (1984). Hypothesis. Vasa vasorum and neovascularization of human coronary arteries: A possible role in the pathophysiology of atherosclerosis. *New England Journal of Medicine, 310,* 175-177.

Barry, W. H., & Grossman, W. (1983). Cardiac catheterization. *New England Journal of Medicine, 309,* 123-125.

Benowitz, N. L. (1988). Nicotine and smokeless tobacco. *CA, 38,* 244-247.

Berger, B. C., & Chung, E. K. (1983). Nuclear cardiology. In E. K. Chung (Ed.), *Quick reference to cardiovascular diseases* (2nd ed., pp. 88-101). Philadelphia: Lippincott.

Best, J. A. (1971). Smoking modification tailored to subject characteristics. *Behavioral Therapy, 2,* 177-191.

Best, J. A. (1975). Tailoring smoking withdrawal procedure to personality and motivation. *Journal of Consultations in Clinical Psychology, 43,* 1-8.

Best, J. A., & Bloch, M. (1979). Compliance in the control of cigarette smoking. In R. B. Haynes, D. W. Taylor, & D. L. Sackett (Eds.), *Compliance in health care* (pp. 202-222). Baltimore: Johns Hopkins University Press.

Bibeau, D. L., Mullen, K. D., McLeroy, K. R., et al. (1988). Evaluations of workplace smoking cessation programs: A critique. *American Journal of Preventive Medicine, 4,* 87-95.

Bjorntorp, P. (1984). Morphological classifications of obesity: What they tell us, what they don't. *International Journal of Obesity, 8,* 523-533.

Borders, C. (Senior Ed.). (1985–1986). A patient care roundtable with patients who had coronary bypass surgery. *Patient Care*

Borders, C. (Senior Ed.). (1985, May). Bypass patients discuss their doctors. *Patient Care,* pp. 46-47. Coronary bypass? Why me?, *Patient Care,* pp. 69-90.

Borders, C. (Senior Ed.). (1985, June). The patient's family confronts bypass. *Patient Care,* pp. 46-63.

Borders, C. (Senior Ed.). (1985, June). Bypass: Patients' perceptions and fears. *Patient Care,* pp. 67-83.

Borders, C. (Senior Ed.). (1985, July). Coronary bypass: 'By God, I made it!'. *Patient Care,* pp. 47-63.

Borders, C. (Senior Ed.). (1985, July). When the bypass patient returns home. *Patient Care,* pp. 65-93.

Borders, C. (Senior Ed.). (1986, Jan.). After bypass: New life, new life-style? *Patient Care,* pp. 111-138.

Borders, C. (Senior Ed.). (1986, Jan.). A doctor discusses his own bypass. *Patient Care,* pp. 141-149.

Bornstein, P. H., Carmody, T. P., Relinger, H., et al. (1977). Reduction of smoking behavior: A multivariate treatment package and the property of response maintenance. *Psychological Records, 27,* 733-741.

Boyd, M. D., & Citro, K. M. (1988, May). Is your MI patient too scared to recover? *RN,* pp. 50-54.

Bray, G. A. (1979). Obesity in America: An overview of the Second Fogarty International Center Conference on Obesity. *International Journal of Obesity, 3,* 363-375.

Breslow, L. (1978). Risk factor intervention for health maintenance. *Science, 200,* 908.

Breu, C. S. (1987). Assessment: Review of vital skills. *In combatting cardiovascular diseases skillfully.* Springhouse, PA: Springhouse Publishing Co.

Society of Actuaries. (1959). *Build and blood pressure study.* Chicago: Author.

Buxton, T., & Pfeffer, J. (1987, Winter). The Healthy People Project: Reducing the risk of heart disease in Maryland. *Journal of Public Health,* pp. 475-490.

Canadian Task Force on the Periodic Examination. (1979). *Task force report.* Ottawa: Canadian Department of National Health and Welfare.

Cantu, R. C. (1980). *Toward physical fitness: Guided exercise for those with health problems.* New York: Human Sciences Press.

Chatterjee, K., Cheitlin, M., Karliner, J., Parmley, W., Rapaport, E., Scheinman, M. (Eds.). (1991). *Cardiology: An illustrated text/reference,* Vol I., Philadelphia, Lippincott.

Carlson, L. A., & Bottinjer, S. (1972). Ischaemic heart disease in relation to fasting values of plasma triglycerides and cholesterol: Stockholm Prospective Study. *Lancet, 1,* 865-868.

Castelli, W. P. (1986). The triglyceride issue: A view from Framington. *American Heart Journal, 112,* 432-437.

Catecholamines in essential hypertension [Editorial]. (1977). *Lancet, 1,* 1088-1090.

Cautela, J. R. (1970). Treatment of smoking by covert sensitization. *Psychological Reports, 26,* 415-420.

Chapman, D., Newcomer, K., Berman, D., et al. (1979). Half-inch vs. quarter-inch Anger camera technology: Resolution and sensitivity difference at low photopak energies. *Journal of Nuclear Medicine, 20,* 610.

Christlieb, A. R. (1973). Diabetes and hypertensive vascular disease: Mechanisms and treatment. *American Journal of Cardiology, 32,* 592-606.

Chung, E. K. (1983a). Ambulatory (Holter monitor) electrocardiography. In E. K. Chung (Ed.), *Quick reference to cardiovascular diseases* (2nd ed pp. 44-56). Philadelphia: Lippincott.

Chung, E. K. (1983b). Exercise (stress) ECG test. In E. K. Chung (Ed.), *Quick reference to cardiovascular diseases* (2nd ed.) (pp. 57-87). Philadelphia: J. P. Lippincott Company.

Chung, E. K. (1986). *Manual of exercise ECG testing.* New York: Yorke Medical Books.

Cohen, S. B. (1988). Tobacco addiction as a psychiatric disease. *Southern Medical Journal, 81,* 1083-1088.

Cohn, J. N., Khatri, I. M., & Hamosh, P. (1970). Bedside catheterization of the left ventricle. *American Journal of Cardiology, 25,* 66.

Colwell, J. A., Lopes-Virella, M., & Halushka, P. V. (1981). Pathogenesis of atherosclerosis in diabetes mellitus. *Diabetes Care, 4,* 121.

Corcoran, D. K. (1988). Helping patients who've had near death experiences. *Nursing 88, 11,* pp. 34-39.

Costa, P. T., Zonderman, A. B., McCrae, R. R., et al. (1983). Content and comprehensiveness in the MMPI: An item factor analysis in a normal adult. *American Journal of Psychiatry, 33,* 47-ff.

Crawley, I. S., Walter, P. F., & Hurst, J. W. (1983). Atherosclerotic heart disease. In E. K. Chung (Ed.), *Quick reference to cardiovascular diseases* (2nd ed pp. 158-173). Philadelphia: Lippincott.

Culpepper, W. S., Sodt, P. C., Messerli, F. H., et al. (1983). Cardiac states in juvenile borderline hypertension. *Annals of Internal Medicine, 98,* 1-7.

Cunningham, R. M., Jr. (1982). *Wellness at work: A report on health and fitness programs for employees of business and industry.* Chicago: Blue Cross and Blue Shield.

Dayton, S., & Pearce, M. L. (1969). Diet high in unsaturated fat: A controlled clinical trial. *Minnesota Medicine, 52*(8), 1237-1242.

DeRisi, W. J., & Butz, G. (1975). *Writing behavioral contracts.* Champaign, IL: Research Press.

Dembrowski, T. M., MacDougall, J. M., Williams, R. B., et al. (1985). Components of type A hostility and angina: A relationship to angiographic findings. *Psychosomatic Medicine, 47,* 219-233.

Dietary guidelines for healthy American adults: A statement for physicians and health professionals by the Nutrition Committee, American Heart Association. (1986). *Circulation, 74,* 1465A-1467A.

Doll, R., & Peto, R. (1976). Mortality in relation to smoking: 20 years observations on male British doctors. *British Medical Journal, 2,* pp. 1525-1536.

Dunbar, J. M., Marshall, G. D., & Hovell, M. F. Behavioral strategies for improving compliance. In R. B. Haynes, D. W. Taylor, & D. L. Sackett (Eds.), *Compliance in health care* (pp. 202-222). Baltimore: Johns Hopkins University Press.

Dunn, F. G., Chandraratra, P., deCarvalho, J. G. R., et al. (1977). Pathophysiologic assessment of hypertensive heart disease with echocardiography. *American Journal of Cardiology, 39,* 789-795.

Dwyer, J., & Mayer, J. (1983). Obesity and coronary heart disease. In R. N. Podell & M. M. Stewart (Eds.), *Primary prevention of coronary heart disease.* Menlo Park, CA: Addison-Wesley.

Edmonson, R. P., Thomas, R. P., Hilton, P. J., et al. (1975). Abnormal leukocyte composition and sodium transport in essential hypertension. *Lancet, 1,* 1003-1009.

Egdahl, R. H., & Goldbeck, W. B. (Eds.) (1980). *Mental wellness programs for employees.* New York: Springer-Verlag.

Eischens, R. R. (1979). Five easy steps for exercise regimen compliance: A new precise guide to running. *Behavioral Medicine, 2,* 14-17.

Elias, J. W., & Marshall, P. H. (Eds.) (1987). *Cardiovascular disease and behavior.* Washington, DC: Hemisphere Publishing .

Eliot, R. S., Buell, J. D., Dembroski, T. M., et al. (1982). Bio-behavioral perspectives on coronary heart disease, hypertension, and sudden cardiac death. *Acta Scandinavia, 660*(Suppl.), 205-213.

Ellestad, M. H. (1986). *Stress testing: Principles and practice* (3rd ed.). Philadelphia: F. A. Davis.

Engel, G. L. (1978). Psychological stress, vasopressor syncope, and sudden death. *Annals of Internal Medicine, 89,* 403-412.

Enos, W. F., Holmes, R. H., & Beyer, J. (1953). Coronary disease among United States soldiers killed in Korea. *Journal of the Americn Medical Association, 152,* 1090-1093.

Everly, G. S., Jr., & Girdano, D. A. (1980). *The stress mess solution* (pp. 121-122). Bowie, MD: Brady Press.

Ewing, J. A. (1984). Detecting alcoholism: The CAGE questionnaire. *Journal of the American Medical Asociation, 252*(14), 1905-1907.

Factor, S., Okun, E., & Minase, T. (1980). Capillary microaneurysms in the human. *New England Journal of Medicine, 302,* 384-388.

Feinlieb, M., Simon, A. B., Gillum, R. F., et al. (1975). Symptoms and signs of sudden death. *Circulation, 51-52* (Suppl. 3), 155-159.

The fifth report of the Joint National Committee on Detection, Evaluation and Treatment of High Blood Pressure. (1993). *Archives of Internal Medicine, 153,* 154-171.

Finnerty, F., Jr. (1981). Hypertension: Specially trained personnel can improve compliance. *Consultant, 21,* 80-90.

Florey, C. du V. (1970). The use and interpretation of ponderal index and other weight-height ratios in epidemiological studies. *Journal of Chronic Diseases, 23,* 93-103.

Flynn, J. B., & Giffin, P. A. (1984). Health promotion in acute care settings. *Nursing Clinics of North America, 19,* 239-250.

Foreman, M. D. (1986). Cardiovascular disease: A men's health hazard. *Nursing Clinics of North America, 21,* 65-71.

Fortmann, S. P., Killen, J. D., Telch, M. J., et al. (1988). Minimal contact treatment for smoking cessation. A placebo controlled trial of nicotine polacrilex and self-directed relapse prevention: Initial results of the Stanford Stop Smoking Project. *Journal of the American Medical Association, 260,* 1575-1580.

Fox, S. M. (1974). *Coronary heart disease: Prevention, detection, rehabilitation, with emphasis on exercise testing.* Denver: International Medical Corporation.

Frankle, R. T., & Yang, M. (Eds.). (1988). *Obesity and weight control: The health professional's guide to understanding and treatment.* Rockville, MD: Aspen.

Friedman, M. (1969). *Pathogenesis of coronary artery disease.* New York: McGraw-Hill.

Friedman, M., & Rosenman, R. H. (1974). *Type A behavior and your heart.* New York: Knopf and Greenwhich, CTL Fawcett.

Frohlich, E. D. (1983). Hypertension and hypertensive heart disease. In E. K. Chung (Ed.), *Quick reference to cardiovascular diseases* (2nd ed., pp. 175-187). Philadelphia: Lippincott.

Fulkerson, P. K. (1985). Echocardiography. In J. W V. Warren & R. P. Lewis (Eds.), *Diagnostic procedures in cardiology: A clinician's guide* (pp. 104-130). Chicago: Year Book Medical.

Garay, R. P., Elghozi, J. L., Dagher, G., et al. (1980). Laboratory distinction between essential and secondary hypertension by measurement of erythrocyte cation fluxes. *New England Journal of Medicine, 302,* 774.

Gatchel, R. J., & Baum, A. (1983). *An introduction to health psychology.* Reading, MA: Addison-Wesley.

Gentry, W. D., & Williams, R. B., Jr. (1979). *Psychological aspects of MI and coronary care.* St. Louis: Mosby.

Getchell, B. (1979). *Physical fitness: A way of life* (2nd ed.). New York: John Wiley & Sons.

Getchell, B. (1980). *Adult physical fitness: A way of life* (pp. 72-73). New York: John Wiley & Sons.

Glantz, S. A., & Parmley, W. W. (1991). Passive smoking and heart disease: Epidemiology, physiology, and biochemistry. *Circulation, 83,* 1-12.

Glasgow, A. M., August, G. P., & Hung, W. (1981). Relationship between control and serum lipids in juvenile-onset diabetes. *Diabetes Care, 4,* 76.

Gotto, A. M., Jr., Bierman, E. L., Connor, W. E., et al. (Eds.). (1984). Recommendations for treatment of hyperlipidemia in adults: A joint statement of the Nutrition Committee and the Council on Arteriosclerosis. Special report. *Circulation, 69,* 1067A-1090A.

Gotto, A. M., Jr., & Wittels, E. H. (1983). Diet, serum cholesterol, lipoproteins, and coronary heart disease: In N. M. Kaplan, & J. Stamler (Eds.), *Prevention of coronary heart disease: Practical management of the risk factors.* Philadelphia: Saunders.

Groszek, E., & Grundy, S. M. (1980). The possible role of the arterial microcirculation in the pathogenesis of atherosclerosis. *Journal of Chronic Diseases, 33,* 679-684.

Grundy, S. M., Greenland, P., Herd, A., et al. (1987). Cardiovascular and risk factor evaluation of healthy American adults: A statement for physicians by an ad hoc committee appointed by the steering committee. *Circulation, 75,* 1339A-1362A.

Gutmann, M. C., & Jackson, T. C. (1987). Facilitating behavior change. In D. P. Sheridan and I. R. Winogrand (Eds.), *The preventive approach to patient care.* New York: Elsevier.

Guzzelta, C. E., & Dossey, B. M. (1984) *Cardiovascular nursing: bodymind tapestry.* St. Louis: Mosby.

Haddy, F. J. (1980). Mechanism, prevention, and therapy in sodium-dependent hypertension. *American Journal of Medicine, 69,* 746-750.

Hall, J. C. (1980). The case for health hazard appraisals: Which health-screening techniques are cost-effective? *Diagnosis, 2,* 60-82.

Hamburg, D. A., Elliott, G. R., & Parron, D. L. (1982). *Health and behavior: Frontiers of research in the biobehavioral sciences.* Washington, DC: National Academy Press.

Hammond, E. C., & Garfinkle, L. (1969). Coronary heart diseases, stroke, and aortic aneurysm: Factors in the etiology. *Archives of Environmental Health, 19,* 167-182.

Hart, J. S. (1967). Commentary on the effect of physical training with and without cold exposure upon physiological indices of fitness for work. *Canadian Medical Association Journal, 96,* 80.

Haynes, S., Feinlieb, M., & Kannel, W. B. (1980). The relationship of psychosocial factors to coronary heart disease in the Framingham study. III. 8-year incidence of CHD. *American Journal of Epidemiology, 111,* 37-58.

Haynes, S., Feinleib, M., Levine, S., et al. (1978). The relationship of psychosocial factors to coronary heart disease in the Framingham study: Prevalence of coronary heart disease. *American Journal of Epidemiology, 107,* 384-402.

Haynes, R. B., Taylor, D. W., & Sackett, D. L. (Eds.). (1980). *Compliance in health care.* Baltimore: Johns Hopkins University Press.

Hazzard, W. L., Goldstein, J. L., Schrott, H. G., et al. (1973). Hyperlipidemia in coronary heart disease: III. Evaluation of lipoprotein phenotypes of 156 genetically defined survivors of myocardial infarction. *Journal of Clinical Investigation, 52,* 1569-1577.

Herje, P. A. (1980). Hows and whys of patient contracting. *Nurse Educator, 5,* 30-34.

Higginbotham, M., Coleman, M., Jones, R. H., et al. (1984). Mechanisms and significance of a decrease in ejection fraction during exercise in patients with coronary artery disease and left ventricular dysfunction at rest. *Journal of the American College of Cardiology, 3,* 88.

Hildebrandt, D. E., & Feldman, S. E. (1975). *The impact of commitment and change tactics training on smoking.* Paper presented at the annual meeting of the Association for Advancement of Behavior Therapy, San Francisco.

Holloway, N. M. (1988). *Nursing the critically ill adult* (3rd Ed.), Menlo Park, CA: Addison-Wesley.

Holme, I., Helgend, A., Hjermann, I., Leven, P., & Lund-Larsen, P. G. (1980). Four-year mortality by some socioeconomic indicators: The Olso study. *Journal of Epidemiology and Community Health, 31*(1), 48-52.

Holmes, T. H., & Rahe, R. H. (1967). The Social Readjustment Rating Scale. *Journal of Psychosomatic Research, 11*(2), 213-218.

Hopkins, P. N., Williams, R. R., & Hunt, S. C. (1984). Magnified risks from cigarette smoking coronary prone families in Utah. *Western Journal of Medicine, 141,* 196-202.

Hubert, H. B., Feinlieb, M., McNamara, P. M., et al. (1983). Obesity as an independent risk factor for heart disease: A 26-year follow-up of participants in the Framingham Heart study. *Circulation, 67,* 968-977.

Hulka, B. S., Cassel, J. C., Kupper, I. I., et al. (1976). Communication, compliance, and concordance between physicians and patients with prescribed medications. *American Journal of Public Health, 48,* 847-853.

Hulley, S. B., Rosenman, R. H., Bawal, J., et al. (1980). Epidemiology as a guide to clinical decisions: The association between triglyceride and coronary heart disease. *New England Journal of Medicine, 302,* 1383-1389.

Hurt, R. D., Offord, K. P., Hepper, N. G., et al. (1988). Long-term follow-up of persons attending a community-based smoking-cessation program. *Mayo Clinic Proceedings, 63,* 681-690.

Hypertension Detection and Follow-up Program Cooperative Group. (1979). Five-year follow-up findings of the hypertension detection and follow-up program. *Journal of the American Medical Association, 242,* 2562.

Isaacs, B., & Kobles, J. (1978). *What it takes to feel good: The Nicholaus technique* (pp. 154-155). New York: Viking Press.

Johnson, J., & Parsons, M. (1984). Symposia on health promotion. *Nursing Clinics of North America, 19,* 195-281.

Kannel, W. B. (1981a). Cigarettes, coronary occlusion, and myocardial infarction. *Journal of the American Medical Association, 246,* 871-872.

Kannel, W. B. (1981b). Update on the role of cigarette smoking in coronary artery disease. *American Heart Journal, 101,* 319- 328.

Kannel, W. B. (1986). Epidemiologic insights into atherosclerotic cardiovascular disease from the Framingham study. In M. L. Pollock and D. H. Schmidt (Eds.), *Heart disease and rehabilitation* (2nd ed., pp. 3-28). New York: John Wiley & Sons.

Kannel, W. B., & Sorlie, P. (1979). Some health benefits of physical activity: The Framingham study. *Archives of Internal Medicine, 139,* 363-375.

Kannel, W. B., Castelli, W. P., & Gordon, T. (1979). Cholesterol in the prediction of atherosclerotic disease: New perspectives based on the Framingham study: *Annals of Internal Medicine, 90,* 85-91.

Kannel, W. B., Sorlie, P., & Gordon, T. (1980). Labile hypertension: A faulty concept. *Circulation, 61,* 1179-1182.

Kannel, W. B. (1989). Risk factors in hypertension. *Journal of Cardiovascular Pharmacology, 13*(Suppl. 1), S4-S10.

Kaplan, N. M. & Lieberman, E. (1990). *Clinical hypertension,.* Baltimore: Williams and Wilkins.

Kaplan, N. M., & Stamler, J. (Eds.). (1983). *Prevention of coronary heart disease: Practical management of the risk factors.* Philadelphia: Saunders.

Kelly, K. L. (1979). Evaluation of a group nutrition education approach to effective internal control. *American Journal of Public Health, 69,* 813-816.

Kerr, C. M., Jr., Reisinger, K. S., & Plankey, F. W. (1978). Sodium concentration of homemade baby foods. *Pediatrics, 62,* 331-335.

Keys, A. (Ed.) (1970). Coronary heart disease in seven countries. *Circulation, 41*(Suppl. I), I1-I8.

Keys, A. (1980). *Seven countries: A multivariate analysis of death and coronary heart disease.* Cambridge, MA: Harvard University Press.

Keys, A., Aravanis, C., Blackburn, H., et al. (1975). Probability of middle-aged men developing coronary heart disease in five years. *Circulation, 45,* 815, 828.

Kimball, C. P. (1981). *The biopsychosocial approach to the patient.* Baltimore: Williams & Wilkins.

Kirkendall, W. M., Feinlab, M., Freis, A., et al. (1980). American Heart Association recommendations for human blood pressure determination by sphygmomanometer. *Circulation, 62,* 1145A-1155A.

Kirscht, J. P., & Rosenstock, I. M. (1979). Patients' problems in following recommendations of health experts. In G. C. Stone, F. Cohen, N. E. Adler, et al. (Eds.), *Health psychology–a handbook: Theories, applications, and challenges of a psychological approach to the health care system* (pp. 189-215). San Francisco: Jossey-Bass.

Klaiber, E. L., Broverman, D. M., Haffajee, C. I., et al. (1982). Serum estrogen levels in men with acute myocardial infarction. *The American Journal of Medicine, 73,* 872-881.

Kleinpell, R. M. (1991). Needs of families of critically ill patients: A literature review. *Critical Care Nurse, 11*(8), 34-40.

Koop, C. E. (1986). An interview with C. Everett Koop, M.D.: Priorities of the Surgeon General. *Nursing Economics, 6,* 107-111.

Koop, C. E. (1988). *Health consequences of smoking.* Washington, DC: National Institutes of Health.

Kramsch, D. M., Aspen, A. J., Abramovitz, B. M., et al. (1981). Reduction of coronary atherosclerosis by moderate conditioning exercise in monkeys on an atherogenic diet. *New England Journal of Medicine, 305,* 1481-1489.

Krtokiewski, M., Bjorntorp, P., Sjostrom, L., et al. (1983). Impact of obesity on metabolism in men and women: Importance of regional adipose tissue distribution. *Journal of Clinical Investigation, 72,* 1150-1160.

Kuller, L. H. (1986). Natural history of coronary heart disease. In M. L. Pollock & D. H. Schmidt (Eds.), *Heart disease and rehabilitation* (2nd ed., pp. 29-51). New York: John Wiley & Sons.

Lapidus, L., Bengtssonn, C., Larsson, B., et al. (1984). Distribution of adipose tissue and risk of cardiovascular disease and death: 12-year follow-up of participants in the population study of Gothenburg, Sweden. *British Medical Journal, 289,* 1257-1261.

Larsson, B., Svardsudd, K., Welin, L., et al. (1984). Abdominal adipose tissue distribution, obesity, and risk of cardiovascular disease and death: A 13-year follow-up of participants in the study of men born in 1913. *British Medical Journal, 288,* 1401-1404.

Lavie, C. J., & Messerli, F. H. (1986). Cardiovascular adaptation to obesity and hypertension. *Chest, 90,* 275-279.

Leon, A. S., & Blackburn, H. (1983). Physical activity. In N. Kaplan & S. Stamler (Eds.), *Prevention of coronary heart disease: Practical management of the risk factors* (pp. 86-97). Philadelphia: Saunders.

Leppo, J., Boucher, C. A., Okada, R. P., et al. (1982). Serum thallium-201 myocardial imaging after dipyridamole infusion: Diagnostic utility in detecting coronary stenoses and relationship to regional wall motion. *Circulation, 66,* 649.

Leventhal, H., & Cleary, P. D. (1986). Behavior modification of risk factors: A problem for a bio-socio-psychological science. In M. L. Pollock & D. H. Schmidt (Eds.), *Heart disease and rehabilitation* (2nd ed., pp. 325-345). New York: John Wiley & Sons.

Levitas, E. L. (1979). Stress testing: New indications, new techniques. *Diagnosis, 1,* 20-29.

Lichtenstein, E., Harris, D. E., Birchler, G. R., et al. (1973). A comparison of rapid smoking, warm, smoking, air, and attention-placebo in the modification of smoking behavior. *Journal of Consulting Clinical Psychology, 40,* 92-98.

Lipid Research Clinics Coronary Primary Prevention Trial Results. I. Reduction in incidence of coronary heart disease. (1984). *Journal of the American Medical Association, 251,* 365.

Lippincott manual of nursing practice (4th ed) (1986). Philadelphia: Lippincott.

Loebel, S., & Spratto, G. (Eds.). (1983). *The nurse's drug handbook.* New York: John Wiley & Sons.

Lorimer, A. S., & Hillis, W. S. (1985). *Cardiovascular disease.* New York: Springer-Verlag.

Loustan, A. (1979, September-October). Using the Health Belief Model to predict patient compliance. *Health Values. Achieving High Level Wellness, 3.*

Luce, B. R., & Schweitzer, S. O. (1978). Smoking and alcohol abuse: A comparison of their economic consequences. *New England Journal of Medicine, 298,* 569-571.

Luria, M. H., Johnson, M. W., Pego, R., et al. (1982). Relationship between sex and hormones: Myocardial infarction and occlusive coronary disease. *Archives of Internal Medicine, 142,* 42-44.Maccoby, N., Farquhar, J. W., Wood, A. J. (1977). Reducing the risk of cardiovascular disease: Effects of a community-based campaign on knowledge and behavior. *Community Health, 2,* 100-114.

Maloney, R. J. (1984). *Hypertension: Risk factors in atherosclerosis. Combatting cardiovascular diseases skillfully.* Springhouse, PA: Springhouse Corporation.

Master, M. A. (1934). Two step test of myocardial function. *American Heart Journal, 10,* 495.

McGee, D., & Gordon, T. (1976). The results of the Framingham study applied to four other U.S.-based epidemiologic studies of cardiovascular disease, section 31. In W. B. Kannel & T. Gordon (Eds.), *The Framingham study: An epidemiologic investigation of cardiovascular disease.* (National Institutes of Health publication No. 76-1083.) Washington, DC: National Heart and Lung Institute.

McGill, H. C. (1968). Fatty streaks in the coronary arteries and aorta. *Laboratory Investigation, 18,* 560-564.

McGill, H. C., Jr., Greer, J. C., & Strong, J. P. (1963). Natural history of human atherosclerotic lesions. In M. Sandler & G. H. Bourne (Eds.), *Atherosclerosis and its origin.* New York: Academic Press.

McGurn, W. C. (1981). *People with cardiac problems: Nursing concepts.* Philadelphia: Lippincott.

Messerli, F. H., Ventura, H., Glade, L. B., et al. (1983). Essential hypertension in the elderly: Haemodynamics, intravascular volume, sodium excretion, and plasma renin activity. *Lancet, 2,* 983-998.

Metropolitan Life Insurance Company. (1983). Metropolitan height and weight tables. *Metropolitan Life Insurance Company Statistical Bulletin, 64,* 1-9.

Miller, D. D., Burns, R. J., Gill, J. B., et al. (Eds.). (1988). *Clinical cardiac imaging.* New York: McGraw-Hill.

Miller, G. J., & Miller, N. E. (1975). Plasma high-density lipoprotein concentration and ischemic heart disease. *Lancet, 1,* 16-19.

Miller, N. E., Thelle, D. S., Forde, O. H., et al. (1977). High-density lipoprotein and coronary heart disease: A prospective case-control study. *Lancet, 1,* 965-968.

Miracle, V. A. (1988). Get in touch and in tune with cardiac assessment, Part 2. *Nursing 88, 18(4),* 41-47.

Morgan, W. P., & Raglin, J. S. (1986). Psychologic aspects of heart disease. In M. L. Pollock and D. H. Schmidt (Eds.), *Heart disease and rehabilitation* (2nd ed., pp. 97-114). New York: John Wiley & Sons.

Moscovitz, J. (1986). *The Rice Diet report: How I lost up to 12 pounds a day on the world-famous weight-loss plan.* New York: Putnam.

Moser, M. (1983). Hypertension and coronary heart disease prevention. In R. N. Podell & M. M. Stewart (Eds.), *Primary prevention of coronary heart disease* (pp. 1-31). Menlo Park, CA: Addison-Wesley.

Multiple Risk Factor Intervention Trial Research Group. (1982). Multiple Risk Factor Intervention Trial: Risk factor changes and mortality results. *Journal of the American Medical Association, 248,* 1465-1477.

Murray, R. B., & Zentner, J. P. (1985). *Nursing assessment and health promotion through the life span.* Englewood Cliffs, NJ: Prentice Hall.

National Center for Health Statistics. (1987). *Exercise and participation in sports among persons 20 years of age and younger.* Washington, DC: U.S. Government Printing Office.

National Heart, Lung, & Blood Institute. (1990). *Morbidity and mortality chartbook on cardiovascular, lung and blood diseases.* Bethesda: Author.

Neaton, J. D., Kuller, L. H., Wentworth, D., et al. (1984). Total and cardiovascular mortality in relation to cigarette smoking, serum cholesterol concentration, and diastolic blood pressure among black and white males followed up for five years (MRFIT). *American Heart Journal, 108,* 759-769.

Neely, E., & Patrick, M. J. (1968). Problems of aged persons taking medications at home. *Nursing Research, 17,* 52-55.

Nimoityn, P., & Chung, E. K. (1983). History taking and physical diagnosis of the cardiovascular system. In E. K. Chung (Ed.), *Quick reference to cardiovascular diseases* (2nd ed., pp. 1-29). Philadelphia: Lippincott.

Novick, L. F., Jillson, D., Coffin, R., et al. (1985). The Vermont Health Risk Survey and the design of community wide preventive health programs. *Journal of Community Health, 10,* 67-80.

Oberman, A., & Naughton, J. (1986). The National Exercise and Heart Disease Project. In M. L. Pollock & D. H. Schmidt (Eds.), *Heart disease and rehabilitation,* (2nd ed., pp. 369-385). New York: John Wiley & Sons.

O'Donnell, M. P., & Ainsworth, T. H. (Eds.). (1984). *Health promotion in the workplace.* New York: John Wiley & Sons.

Okene, J. K., Aney, J., Goldberg, R. J., et al. (1988). A survey of Massachusetts physicians' smoking intervention practices. *American Journal of Preventive Medicine, 4,* 14-20.

Osler, W. (1910). Lumleian lectures. *Lancet, 1,* 687, 839, 973.

Pakrashi, B. C., Demany, M. A., & Zimmerman, H. A. (1983). Cardiac catheterization and coronary arteriography. In E. K. Chung (Ed.), *Quick reference to cardiovascular diseases* (2nd ed., pp. 136-157). Philadelphia: Lippincott.

Paffenberger, R. S., Jr. (1986). Exercise in the primary prevention of coronary heart disease. In M. L. Pollock & D. H. Schmidt (Eds.), *Heart disease and rehabilitation* (2nd ed., pp. 349-368). New York: John Wiley & Sons.

Paffenberger, R. S., Jr., & Hale, W. E. (1975). Work activity and coronary heart mortality. *New England Journal of Medicine, 292,* 545-550.

Paffenberger, R. S., Jr., Laughlin, M. E., Gima, A. S., et al. (1978). Physical activity as an index of heart attack risk in college alumni. *American Journal of Epidemiology, 108,* 161-175.

Pender, N. J. (1987). *Health promotion in nursing practice.* Norwalk, CT: Appleton-Century-Crofts.

Perper, J. A., Kuller, L. H., & Cooper, M. (1975). Coronary arteries in sudden, unexpected deaths. In R. J. Prineus & H. Blackburn (Eds.), *Sudden coronary death outside the hospital* (pp. 27-33). Dallas: American Heart Association.

Phillips, G. B., Kastelli, W. P., Abbott, R. P., & McNamara, P. M. (1983). Association of hyperestrogenemia and coronary heart disease in men in the Framingham cohort. *Archives of Internal Medicine, 74,* 863-869.

Phillips, N. R., Havel, R. J., & Kane, J. P. (1981). Levels and interrelationships of serum and lipoprotein cholesterol and triglycerides: Association with adiposity and the consumption of ethanol, tobacco, and beverages containing caffeine. *Arteriosclerosis, 1,* 13-24.

Pierce, J. P., Fiore, M. C., Novotny, T. E., et al. (1989). Trends in cigarette smoking in the United States: Projections to the year 2000. *Journal of the American Medical Association, 261,* 61-65.

Podell, R. N. (1983). The Multiple Risk Factor Intervention Trial (MRFIT): Summary of findings and preliminary interpretation, September 1982. In R. N. Podell & M. M. Stewart (Eds.), *Primary prevention of coronary heart disease: A practical guide for the clinician* (pp. 326-334). Menlo Park, CA: Addison-Wesley.

Podell, R. N., & Stewart, M. M. (Eds.). (1983). *Primary prevention of coronary heart disease: A practical guide for the clinician.* Menlo Park, CA: Addison-Wesley Publishing Company.

Pooling Project Research Group. (1978). Relationship of blood pressure, serum cholesterol, smoking habit, relative weight, and ECG abnormalities to incidence of major coronary events: Final report of the Pooling Project. *Journal of Chronic Diseases, 31,* 201-306.

Poston, L., Sewell, R. B., Wilkinson, S. P., et al. (1981). Evidence for a circulatory sodium transport inhibitor in essential hypertension. *British Medical Journal, 282,* 847-849.

Rankin, S. H., & Duffy, K. L. (1983). *Patient education: Issues, principles, and guidelines.* Philadelphia: Lippincott.

Rankin, S. H. (1992). Psychosocial adjustments of coronary artery disease patients and their spouses: Nursing implications. *Nursing Clinics of North America, 27*(1), 271-284.

Redman, B. K. (1981). *Issues and concepts in patient education.* New York: Appleton-Century-Crofts.

Reubi, R. C., Weidmann, P., Hodler, J., et al. (1978). Changes in neural function with essential hypertension. *American Journal of Medicine, 64,* 556-563.

Rogot, E., & Murray, J. L. (1980). Smoking and causes of death among U.S. veterans: 16 years of observation. *Public Health Reports, 95,* 213-222.

Rorden, J. W. (1987). *Nurses as health teachers: A practical guide.* Philadelphia: Saunders.

Rosenman, R. H., & Chesney, M. A. (1983). Type A behavior pattern and coronary heart disease. In R. N. Podell & M. M. Stewart (Eds.), *Primary prevention of coronary heart disease: A practical guide for the clinician* (pp. 172-196). Menlo Park, CA: Addison-Wesley.

Rosenman, R. H., & Friedman, M. (1974). Neurogenic factors in pathogenesis of coronary heart disease. *Medical Clinics of North America, 58,* 269-279.

Rosenman, R. H., Friedman, M., Straus, R., et al. (1964). The Western Collaborative Group Study. *Journal of the American Medical Association, 189,* 15-22.

Rosenstock, I. M. (1960). What research in motivation suggests for public health. *American Journal of Public Health, 50*(3), 295-302.

Rosenstock, I. M. (1966). Why people use health services. *Milbank Memorial Fund Quarterly, 44,* 94-124.

Ross, R. (1986). The pathogenesis of atherosclerosis: An update. *New England Journal of Medicine, 314,* 488-500.

Rotter, J. B. (1971). *Clinical psychology.* Englewood Cliffs, NJ: Prentice-Hall.

Sackett, D., Haynes, R., Gibson, E., et al. (1978). Patient compliance with antihypertensive regimes. *Patient Counseling and Health Education, 1,* 18-21.

Salonen, J. T., Puska, P., & Tuomilehto, J. (1982). Physical activity and risk of myocardial infarction, cerebral stroke, and death: A longitudinal study in Eastern Finland. *American Journal of Epidemiology, 115,* 526-537.

Saltykow, S. (1975). Jegenoliche und beginnende atherosklerse. *Coronary Bulletin of the Swiss Arts, 45,* 1057.

Savage, D. D., Drager, J. I. M., & Henry, W. L. (1979). Echocardiographic assessment of cardiac anatomy and function in hypertension patients. *Circulation, 59,* 623-632.

Scherer, D., & Kaltenbach, M.: (1979). Frequency of life-threatening complications associated with stress testing. *Deutsche Medizinische Wochenschrift, 104,* 116.

Sempos, C., Cooper, R., Kovar, M. G., et al. (1988). Divergence of the recent trends in coronary mortality for the four major race-sex groups in the United States. *American Journal of Public Health, 78,* 1422-1427.

Severson, H. H., & Hynd, G. W. (1977). A comparison of the effectiveness of rapid smoking, modeling, and covert sensitization in smoking cessation. Paper presented at the annual meeting of the Western Psychological Association, Seattle.

Shephard, R. J. (1983). Exercise and primary prevention of coronary heart disease. In R. N. Podell & M. M. Stewart (Eds.). *Primary prevention and coronary heart disease: A practical guide for the clinician.* Menlo Park, CA: Addison-Wesley.

Sheridan, D. P., & Winogrond, I. R. (Eds.). (1987). *The preventive approach to patient care.* New York: Elsevier.

Shipley, R. H., Orleans, C. T., Wilbur, C. S., et al. (1988). Effect of the Johnson & Johnson Live for Life program on employee smoking. *Preventive Medicine, 17,* 25-34.

Simonson, M., & Heilman, J. R. (1983). *The complete university medical diet.* New York: Rawson Associates.

Smilkstein, G., Ashworth, C., & Montano, D. (1982). Validity and reliability of the Family APGAR as a test of family function. *Journal of Family Medicine, 15*(2), 303-311.

Smitherman, C. (1981). Your patient's angry–what should you do? *Nursing 81, 11,* 96-97.

Sones, F. M., & Shirey, E. K. (1962). Cine coronary arteriography. *Modern Concepts in Cardiovascular Disease, 31,* 735.

Sokolow, M., McIlroy, M. B., & Cheitlin, M. D. (1990). *Clinical cardiology.* Norwalk, CT: Appleton and Lange.

Sports medicine for children and youth. (1979). Columbus, OH: Ross Laboratories.

Stamler, J. (1983). Nutrition-related risk factors for the atherosclerotic diseases: Present status. *Progress in Biochemical Pharmacology, 19,* 245-308.

Steptoe, A., & Mathews, A. (Eds.). (1984). *Health care and human behavior.* Orlando: Academic Press.

Strong, W. B. (1983). Atherosclerosis: Its pediatric roots. In N. M. Kaplan & J. Stamler (Eds.), *Prevention of coronary heart disease: Practical management of the risk factors* (pp. 20-32). Philadelphia: Saunders.

Suitor, C. W., & Hunter, M. F. (1980). *Principles and application in health promotion* (pp. 425-434). Philadelphia: Lippincott.

Tei, C., & Shah, P. M. (1983). Echocardiography. In E. K. Chung (Ed.), *Quick reference to cardiovascular diseases* (2nd ed., p. 140). Philadelphia: Lippincott.

Thelan, L. A., Davie, J. K., & Viden, L. D. (1990).*Textbook of critical care nursing.* St. Louis: Mosby.

Thomas, H. E., Jr., & Kannel, W. B. (1986). Risk factors for coronary heart disease. In E. K. Chung (Ed.), *Quick reference to cardiovascular diseases* (2nd ed., pp. 44-56). Philadelphia: Lippincott.

Thompson, E. B., Hamrell, M., & Coffin, R. R. (1987, Spring). The Heart Healthy Vermonter Program. *Journal of Public Health Policy,* pp. 36-43.

Thomson. P., & Kelemen, M. H. (1975). Hypotension accompanying the onset of exertional angina. *Circulation, 52,* 28.

Tirrell, B. E., & Hart, L. K. (1980). The relationship of health beliefs and knowledge to exercise compliance in patients after coronary bypass. *Heart & Lung, 9(3),* 487-493.

Turpeinen, O., Karvonen, M. J., Pekkarinen, M., et al. (1979). Dietary prevention of coronary heart disease: The Finnish Mental Hospital Study. *International Journal of Epidemiology, 8,* 99-118.

Underhill, S., Woods, S., Sivarajan Froelicher, C., & Halpenny, C. (1990). *Cardiovascular medications for cardiac nursing.* Philadelphia: Lippincott.

U.S. Department of Health, Education, and Welfare. (1979). *Health consequences of smoking: Cardiovascular diseases: A report of the Surgeon General.* Washington, DC: U.S. Government Printing Office.

Vanderschmidt, H. F., Koch-Weser, D., & Woodbury, P. A. (1987). *Handbook of clinical prevention.* Baltimore: Wiliams & Wilkins.

Veterans' Administration Cooperative Study Group. (1967). Effects of treatment on morbidity in hypertension. *Journal of the American Medical Association, 202,* 1028-1034.

Veterans' Administration Cooperative Study Group. (1970). Effects of treatment on morbidity in hypertension: Results in patients with diastolic blood pressure averaging 90 through 114 mm Hg. *Journal of the American Medical Association, 213,* 1143-1152.

Veterans Administration Cooperative Study Group on Antihypertensive Agents. (1972). Effects of treatment on morbidity in hypertension. III. Influence of age, diastolic pressure, and prior cardiovascular disease: Further analysis of side effects. *Circulation, 45,* 991.

Wald, N. J., Howard, S., Smith, P. G., et al. (1973). Association between atherosclerotic diseases and carboxyhemoglobin levels in tobacco smokers. *British Medical Journal, 1,* 761-763.

Waldron, I., Zyzanski, S., Skekelle, R., et al. (1977). The coronary-prone behavior pattern in employed men and women. *Journal of Human Stress,* 2-18.

Warren, J. V., & Lewis, R. P. (Eds.). (1985). *Diagnostic procedures in cardiology: A clinician's guide.* Chicago: Year Book Medical.

Watkins, H. H. (1976). Hypnosis and smoking: A five-session approach. *International Journal of Clinical and Experimental Hypnosis, 24,* 381-390.

Wells, A. (1990). An estimate of adult mortality in the U. S. from passive smoke: Response to criticism. *Environmental International, 16,* 187-193.

Wenger, N. K. (1983). Exercise prescription for patients with coronary disease and for healthy individuals. In E. K. Chung (Ed.), *Quick reference to cardiovascular diseases* (2nd ed., pp. 30-39). Philadelphia: J. P. Lippincott.

Wenger, N. K. (Ed.). (1985). *Exercise and the heart* (2nd ed.) Philadelphia: F. A. Davis.

Williams, R. B. (1984). Neuroendocrine response patterns and stress: Biobehavioral mechanisms of disease. In R. B. Williams (Ed.), *Perspectives on behavioral medicine: Neuroendocrine control and behavior.* New York: Academic Press.

Williams, R. R., Hunt, S. C., Barlow, G. K., et al. (1988). Health family trees: A tool for finding and helping young family members of coronary and cardiac prone pedigrees in Texas and Utah. *American Journal of Public Health, 78,* 1283-1286.

Woldrum, K. M., Ryan-Morrell, V., Towson, M. C., et al. (1985). *Patient education: Foundations of practice.* Rockville, MD: Aspen.

Wolf, R. N., & Grundy, S. M. (1983). Influence of weight reduction on plasma lipoproteins in obese patients. *Arteriosclerosis, 3,* 160-169.

Wood, P. D., Stefanick, M. L., Dreon, D. M., et al. (1988). Changes in plasma lipids and lipoproteins in overweight men during weight loss through dieting as compared with exercise. *New England Journal of Medicine, 319,* 1173-1179.

Wood, P. P., Haskell, W., Stern, M. P., et al. (1977). Plasma lipoprotein distribution in male and female runners. *Annals of the New York Academy of Science, 301,* 748, 763.

Working Group on Arteriosclerosis of the National Heart, Lung, and Blood Institute. (1981). Vol. 2. (NIH Publication No. 81-2035.) Bethesda: U.S. Department of Health and Human Services.

The world almanac and book of facts. (1988). New York: Scripps Howard Co.

Zifferblatt, S. M. (1983). Health habits and behavior change: Realigning expectations in reality. In R. N. Podell & M. M. Stewart (Eds.), *Primary prevention of coronary heart disease.* Menlo Park, CA: Addison-Wesley.

Zinner, S. H., Margolius, H. S., Rosner, B., et al. (1978). Stability of blood pressure rank and urinary kallikrein concentration in childhood: An 8-year follow-up. *Circulation, 58,* 908-915.

GLOSSARY

Aneurysm - A localized abnormal dilatation of a blood vessel. Usually due to a congenital defect or weakness of the wall of the vessel.

Angina pectoris - Pain radiating from the heart due to a lack of oxygen and blood supply, often characterized by a feeling of suffocation, chest pain, jaw or shoulder pain.

Anorexia - Abnormal lack or loss of appetite.

Apical - The area pertaining to the apex, which is the summit or highest point of an object.

Arrhythmias - Abnormal heart rhythms.

Arteriogram - An radiographic study of the function and anatomy of an artery.

Asymptomatic - Without any symptoms or complaints

Atheroma - Fatty degeneration or thickening of the wall of the larger arteries.

Atherosclerosis - Accumulations of lipid or fatty material within the lining of blood vessels. Leads to narrowing of the arteries.

Atrophy - The reduction in size of a structure such as a muscle.

Aversion - A strong desire to avoid because of dislike.

Awareness - A patient's realization there is something wrong with his or her heart.

Behavioral contract - An agreement by a patient with a health care provider to follow a prescribed plan designed to improve the patient's health status.

Biofeedback - A relaxation technique used to manage or reduce stress.

Body mass index (BMI) - Weight (in kilograms) divided by height (in meters) squared (wt/ht^2).

Cardiac catheterization - A test done to evaluate the function and pressures of the heart. A catheter is inserted into a large vein and passed first into the right atrium, through the right ventricle, and finally into the pulmonary artery. The catheter may be left in place for a period of days to continuously evaluate heart function.

Catabolized - The destructive phase of metabolism in which complex substances are broken down to simpler substances.

Chronologic - Occurring in sequence from earliest to latest.

Claudication - Lameness or limping often caused by inadequate blood supply in the lower leg or calf area.

Clubbing of the fingers - Rounding of ends and swelling of fingers often due to heart or lung disease.

Coarctation - Compression or narrowing of the walls of a vessel.

Collagen - A fibrous insoluble protein found in connective tissue.

Compliance - Following the prescribed plan of care.

Congenital defects - Abnormalities or deformities present at birth.

Control - A real or perceived ability to determine the outcome of an event.

Coronary angiography - A test done to evaluate the circulation of the arteries of the heart. A catheter is inserted, usually into the femoral artery, and passed up to the origin of the coronary arteries where radiologic contrast material is injected while pictures of the heart are taken to outline the arteries with the contrast material flowing through them.

Coronary bypass grafting - A surgical procedure in which diseased and narrowed arteries of the heart are provided with new blood circulation by the use of vein grafts or other arteries.

Cyanosis - Bluish discoloration of the skin due to reduced amounts of hemoglobin in the circulating blood.

Denial - Refusing to believe something, such as a patient not believing he or she has had a heart attack.

Depression - A common mental state for a patient after a heart attack. Signs and symptoms include disinterest, increased sleep patterns, and a sense of doom.

Dissection - Cutting into a part of a vessel, causing damage and a potential obstruction or lack of blood flow.

Diabetic microangiopathy - Disease of the smaller blood vessels due to diabetes mellitus.

Digital subtraction angiography (DSA) - A test done to determine the function of the chambers and valves of the heart. Radiologic contrast material is injected through a vein, and radiographs are taken to visualize the contrast material in the heart structures.

Dysrhythmias - Abnormal heart rhythms.

Dyspnea - Difficulty breathing or shortness of breath.

Echocardiography - A test used to evaluate the structures and function of the heart by sending and recording sound waves.

Ejection fraction - The amount of blood that is ejected from the heart with each heart beat or contraction. Usually reported as a percentage. Normal is 50–65%.

Empathetic - Identification with the feelings of another person. Understanding how another might feel or behave.

Endurance exercise - Vigorous activity that involves the large muscles of the body.

Euphoria - Heightened inner awareness and increased feelings of self-control.

Exacerbate - To make worse. Aggravation of signs or symptoms leading to an increase in the severity of a disease.

Exercise prescription - A medical plan of specific activities and exercise.

Goiter - Enlargement of the thyroid often due to an infection or tumor.

Hemoptysis - Coughing or spitting up blood from the lungs, trachea, bronchi, or larynx.

Hyperglycemia - An elevation of the glucose level in the blood.

Hypertrophy - Abnormal enlargement of a body part or organ.

ICU psychosis - The confusion or disorientation a patient experiences after being in an ICU for a period. Often due to lack of sleep, sensory stimulation, or effects of medication.

Kallikrein - A enzyme found in blood plasma, urine, and body tissues. When activated, one of the most potent vasodilators.

Ketoacidosis - An acid-base disturbance resulting in an excess amount of acids caused by an abnormal breakdown of fat molecules.

Learned helplessness - A condition that develops when a person cannot gain a sense of control over what happen to him or her.

Lipoprotein - Simple proteins combined with lipid components such as cholesterol, triglycerides, and phospholipid.

Magnetic resonance imaging (MRI) - A test used to evaluate heart function through the use of strong magnetic forces that generate images of the heart and its structures.

Metabolic equivalent unit (MET) - The energy required to perform a specific action, based on the amount of oxygen consumed at 3.5 ml/kg per minute.

Murmur - A soft blowing or rasping sound heard on auscultation of the heart or a large artery.

Myocardial imaging - A test used to detect areas of infarcted heart muscle inwhich isotopes are injected into the patient's blood and then a scan is obtained of the heart to isolate areas of infarcted muscle.

Myocarditis - Infliction of the heart muscle.

Noncompliance - Inability or unwillingness to follow a prescribed plan. A patient not following doctor's orders.

Obesity - Abnormal amount of fat on the body. Usually means the person is more than 30% over the average weight for his or her height, age, and sex.

Overweight - Weighing more than is generally accepted to be normal.

Pallor - Pale skin or lack of color.

Palpitations - An uncomfortable or strange feeling in the chest often described as a racing heart beat or skipping beats.

Pansystolic murmur - A murmur of the heart heard during all of the period of systole.

Patent ductus arteriosus - An open channel of communication between the main pulmonary artery and the aorta.

Pericarditis - Inflammation of the protective sac around the heart.

Photophobia - Unusual intolerance to light.

Placebo - A inactive substance having no medicinal value but given to a patient who believes it will have an effect or cure.

Positive emission tomography (PET) - A test used to determine areas of healthy and infarcted heart muscle in which isotopes are injected into the patient's blood and taken up in the heart muscle.

Primary prevention - Intervening to change risks before disease or illness occurs. To delay or prevent the onset of illness by detecting and altering high risk behavior.

Primary risk factors - Conditions that directly increase the patient's risk for a disease.

Psychoneurotic - Disturbances in thought, attitudes, behavior, and feelings related to emotional conflict.

Pulse pressure - The difference between the systolic and diastolic blood pressure. For example if systole = 130 and diastole = 80, then pulse pressure = 50.

Pulsus alternans - A pulse that consistently alternates from strong to weak beats.

Pulsus paradoxus - A pulse that becomes weaker on inspiration.

Pyelogram - A radiograph of the ureter and renal pelvis.

Reinforcement - Encouraging or promoting positive behavior.

Sedentary - Inactive or leading a lifestyle that is characterized by little or no physical activity.

Self-contract - A commitment made by a person to himself or herself to perform specific behaviors for previously determined reinforcement that is both attractive and motivating.

Self-monitoring - The process of observing and recording one's own behavior.

Stenosis - Narrowing or constriction of a passage or orifice.

Synergistic - The joint action of drugs that when taken together increase each other's effectiveness.

Syncope - A transitory loss of consciousness caused by inadequate blood flow to the brain.

Thallium - A metallic element injected into the blood to look for abnormalities of blood distribution with the use of x-rays.

Thromboembolism - A blood clot that is travelling within the circulation causing obstruction of blood flow to an area.

Thrombus - A blood clot obstructing a blood vessel or a chamber of the heart.

Transfer anxiety - A state of uneasiness and concern over being moved from the ICU to a less acute area.

Type A personality - The type of person characterized by competitiveness, impatience, intense drive and desire to achieve, and a sense of urgency.

Valsalva maneuver - Holding one's breath and bearing down, which leads to increased intrathoracic pressure.

INDEX

PRETEST KEY

1.	A	Chapter 1
2.	A	Chapter 1
3.	B	Chapter 1
4.	A	Chapter 1
5.	C	Chapter 3
6.	A	Chapter 3
7.	B	Chapter 4
8.	B	Chapter 4
9.	B	Chapter 4
10.	B	Chapter 4
11.	B	Chapter 5
12.	D	Chapter 5
13.	C	Chapter 5
14.	B	Chapter 6
15.	A	Chapter 6
16.	D	Chapter 6
17.	B	Chapter 6
18.	B	Chapter 7
19.	A	Chapter 7
20.	B	Chapter 7
21.	A	Chapter 8
22.	B	Chapter 8
23.	A	Chapter 8
24.	C	Chapter 8
25.	D	Chapter 9

NOTES

NOTES